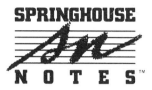

GUIDE TO SURVIVING NURSING SCHOOL

Joan M. Regan, RN, MSN

Ms. Regan, the author of this book, is an Instructor of Nursing at Quincy (Massachusetts) Junior College. She earned her BSN from the University of Rhode Island at Kingston, and her MSN from Boston University. Ms. Regan is a member of the American Nurses' Association and the Massachusetts Nurses' Association. She is a past member of the District V Nursing Practice Committee, and is currently a member of the Council on Nursing Education.

Joanne Trekas, ARNP, PhD

Dr. Trekas, the reviewer of this book, is Director of the Nursing Division at the University of Tampa, Florida. She earned her BSN and MSN from the University of Wisconsin at Milwaukee, and her PhD from Marquette University. Dr. Trekas is a member of the American Nurses' Association, the Florida Nurses' Association, the National League for Nursing, and Sigma Theta Tau.

Springhouse Corporation
Springhouse, Pennsylvania

Staff

Executive Director, Editorial
Stanley Loeb

Director of Trade and Textbooks
Minnie B. Rose, RN, BSN, MEd

Art Director
John Hubbard

Clinical Consultant
Maryann Foley, RN, BSN

Senior Acquisitions Editor
Susan L. Mease

Editor
Kate Cassidy

Copy Editor
Mary Hohenhaus Hardy

Designers
Stephanie Peters (associate art director),
Susan Hopkins Rodzewich

Art Production
Robert Perry (manager), Heather Bernhardt,
Anna Brindisi, Donald Knauss, Tom Robbins,
Robert Wieder

Typography
David Kosten (director), Diane Paluba (manager),
Joyce Rossi Biletz, Elizabeth Bergman, Phyllis
Marron, Robin Rantz, Valerie L. Rosenberger

Manufacturing
Deborah Meiris (manager), T.A. Landis,
Jennifer Suter

Production Coordination
Aline S. Miller (manager), Maura Murphy

Library of Congress Cataloging-in-Publication Data

Regan, Joan M.
 Guide to surviving nursing school / Joan M. Regan, author; Joanne Trekas, reviewer.
  p. cm. — (Springhouse notes)
 Includes bibliographical references.
 Includes index.
 ISBN 0-87434-316-X
 1. Nursing—Study and teaching. 2. Nursing students—Psychology.
 I. Trekas, Joanne. II. Title. III. Series.
  [DNLM: 1. Curriculum. 2. Education, Nursing.
 3. Students, Nursing—psychology. WY 18
 R333g] RT73.R35   1991
 610.73'071'1—dc20
 DNLM/DLC   90-10

Contents

How to Use Springhouse Notes

Today, more than ever, nursing students face enormous time pressures. Nursing education has become more sophisticated, increasing the difficulties students have with studying efficiently and keeping pace.

The need for a comprehensive, well-designed series of study aids is great, which is why we've produced Springhouse Notes...to meet that need. Springhouse Notes provide essential course material in outline form, enabling the nursing student to study more effectively, improve understanding, achieve higher test scores, and get better grades.

Key features appear throughout each book, making the information more accessible and easier to remember.
- **Learning Objectives.** These objectives precede each section in the book to help the student evaluate knowledge before and after study.
- **Key Points.** Highlighted in color throughout the book, these points provide a way to quickly review critical information. Key points may include:
  —a cardinal sign or symptom of a disorder
  —the most current or popular theory about a topic
  —a distinguishing characteristic of a disorder
  —the most important step of a process
  —a critical assessment component
  —a crucial nursing intervention
  —the most widely used or successful therapy or treatment.
- **Points to Remember.** This information, found at the end of each section, summarizes the section in capsule form.
- **Glossary.** Difficult, frequently used, or sometimes misunderstood terms are defined for the student at the end of each section.

Remember: Springhouse Notes are learning tools designed to *help* you. They are not intended for use as a primary information source. They should never substitute for class attendance, text reading, or classroom note-taking.

This book, *Guide to Surviving Nursing School,* addresses the common concerns of students entering or reentering a nursing education program. Important topics covered include registration and course selection, classroom skills, financial assistance, time management, stress management, curriculum content, study skills, clinical learning, and test taking. The book also deals with life after graduation, providing information on coping with transition, obtaining a license, job hunting, and continuing education. It concludes with practical advice on how to succeed in professional nursing.

Getting Started

Learning Objectives

After studying this section, the reader should be able to:

- Identify the factors that influence the choice of nursing as a career.

- Describe the education programs that lead to a career in nursing.

- Discuss factors to consider when choosing a nursing education program.

- Present strategies for adjusting to a nursing education program.

I. Getting Started

A. Introduction

1. The choice of nursing as a career is influenced by personal characteristics and the types of education programs available
2. Personal characteristics that lead to an interest in nursing include:
   a. Desire to help others
   b. Belief in the value of individuals to society
   c. Interest in science
   d. Interest in social sciences
   e. Interest in health care
   f. Respect for the profession
3. Types of education programs available vary, depending on geographic location
4. Basic registered nursing programs available (see *Comparing nursing education programs*) include:
   a. Diploma program
   b. Bachelor of Science in Nursing (BSN) degree program
   c. Associate degree (AD) program
5. Nursing programs share several characteristics
   a. All graduates take the National Council Licensure Examination for Registered Nurses (NCLEX-RN)
   b. All graduates must achieve a minimum score to pass the test and become licensed
   c. After passing the test, graduates may use the title of Registered Nurse
   d. All schools must meet the criteria established for state board approval and national accreditation
6. Diploma programs are the oldest type of nursing education, first developed in the late 1800s
   a. Developed to staff hospitals by training students there and having them practice there after graduation
   b. Experienced decreased enrollments as students elected to seek a college degree
7. Characteristics of a diploma nursing program include:
   a. Affiliation with a hospital
   b. Duration of 18 to 36 months
   c. Concentration on nursing courses and applying knowledge to patient care
   d. In some cases, affiliation with local college, where students take science courses at the college and transfer credits
   e. Presentation of a diploma in nursing to the graduating student who is then eligible to take the NCLEX-RN

8. BSN programs date to the early 1900s
   a. BSN programs were developed to provide nurses with a broad-based education
   b. Early BSN programs lasted 5 years, providing 2 years of liberal arts education and 3 years of basic nursing education
9. Characteristics of BSN programs include:
   a. Operation from a private or public college or university
   b. Usual duration of 4 academic years
   c. Concentration on general education courses, including English, the humanities, and the behavioral, natural, and social sciences, and on nursing courses
   d. Presentation of a BSN to the graduating student who is then eligible to take the NCLEX-RN
10. AD programs were developed in the 1950s as a response to the post-World War II nursing shortage
   a. AD programs were developed to train *technical nurses*; however, that term has not been defined clearly
   b. Growth has paralleled that of community colleges in the United States
11. Characteristics of an AD programs include:
   a. Operation from a junior or community college
   b. Usual duration of 2 academic years
   c. Presentation of general and nursing courses
   d. Presentation of an AD in nursing to the graduating student, who is then eligible to take the NCLEX-RN
12. The nurse who completes a basic education program and attains a license may seek additional academic degrees
   a. Licensed Practical Nurse (LPN) to RN (AD): length of program varies; advanced placement is possible; usually offered at a community college

COMPARING NURSING EDUCATION PROGRAMS

This chart compares the three basic types of nursing education programs.

TYPE OF PROGRAM	CHARACTERISTICS
Diploma	• 18 to 36 months • hospital-based • may or may not award college credits
AD	• 2 years • community college- or junior college-based • 60 college credits awarded
BSN	• 4 years • college- or university-based • 120 college credits awarded

    b. RN (Diploma or AD) to BSN: length of program varies; offered at a college or university

    c. RN (BSN) to Master's degree: length of program varies from 1 to 3 years; offered at a college or university

    d. Master's degree to Doctoral program: length of program varies; offered at a college or university (For more information on advanced education, see Section XV-H)

13. When choosing an education program, the student must consider many factors

    a. Career goals

    b. Age

    c. Motivation

    d. Program cost and personal financial resources

    e. Program availability

    f. Personal circumstances and responsibilities

    g. Employment obligations

    h. Work experience

    i. Educational background

14. At one time, most nursing students were recent high school graduates; today's entering students have widely varied backgrounds

15. Today's nursing students may have to cope not only with the demands of the education program, but also with larger responsibilities and commitments

16. All nursing students must develop *survival strategies* to help them succeed

    a. Know the curriculum plan; course prerequisites, scheduling, and sequencing; and credit requirements

    b. Become familiar with the campus, including the library, computer and science laboratories, health services, financial resources, and learning resources

    c. Develop and maintain a beneficial relationship with the academic advisor

    d. Develop classroom skills, including listening and note-taking

    e. Develop study skills

    f. Develop communication skills

    g. Develop examination-taking skills

    h. Develop time-management skills

    i. Develop stress-management skills

17. These survival strategies can be used by anyone entering nursing school, including recent high school graduates, those who have been away from school for many years, LPNs, and RNs reentering school

B. Recent high school graduate entering nursing

1. Student characteristics

    a. Typically age 18

    b. Limited in experience in health care

    c. Usually without family obligations

       d. Interested in establishing a career
       e. Interested in socializing with other students
       f. Interested in experiencing college life
       g. Interested in becoming independent
       h. Accustomed to a directed, structured learning environment

2. Problems encountered in adjusting to nursing school
       a. Managing time in an unstructured environment
       b. Adjusting to independence
       c. Balancing social activities with study demands
       d. Adjusting to being away from home

3. Survival strategies
       a. Manage time efficiently to avoid additional stress
       b. Become familiar with course prerequisites, scheduling, and sequencing, and credit requirements, to assist with planning
       c. Get to know academic advisor and maintain contact throughout the program to help with adjustment
       d. Set priorities and organize tasks to balance academic demands with personal and social life

C. Entering nursing after years away from school
1. Student characteristics
       a. Typically age 20 or older
       b. Interest in establishing or advancing in a career or in changing careers
       c. Strong motivation
       d. Goal-directed
       e. Possible family and employment responsibilities

2. Problems encountered in adjusting to nursing school
       a. Age difference; may be older than classmates
       b. Feelings of inadequacy from having been away from school
       c. Role conflict among family, employment, school and social demands
       d. Insufficient study skills
       e. Unfamiliarity with course prerequisites, scheduling, and sequencing and with credit requirements
       f. Inefficient use of time

3. Survival strategies
       a. Improve study and note-taking skills
       b. Become familiar with course prerequisites, scheduling, and sequencing and with credit requirements to assist with planning
       c. Get to know academic advisor and maintain contact throughout the program to assist with problems and adjustment
       d. Allow extra time for studying
       e. Be positive about work and life experiences to prevent feelings of inadequacy

    f. When appropriate, share work and life experiences in class to enhance self-esteem

    g. Equate age with experience and consider it an asset

    h. Participate in class; avoid isolation from other students

    i. Be self-confident and assertive, but do not overcompensate by monopolizing the class

    j. Treat other students as peers; do not patronize them

    k. Evaluate family, employment, personal, and social obligations to plan for all demands on time

    l. Develop a time-management plan, making study a priority

    m. Know limitations; take on only responsibilities that can be handled without overloading the schedule

    n. Expect disruptions in life-style; make necessary adjustments

D. LPN entering nursing

  1. Student characteristics

    a. May be any age

    b. Experience in health care

    c. Experience in structured nursing program

    d. Previous skill-oriented learning in nursing

    e. Desire for professional status

    f. Goal-directed

    g. Possible family and employment responsibilities

  2. Problems encountered in adjusting to nursing school

    a. Possible need to repeat courses

    b. Conflict between school values and work values

    c. Unfamiliarity with course prerequisites, scheduling, and sequencing and with credit requirements

    d. Time management

    e. Feelings of superiority to other students because of previous learning or work experience

    f. Transition to a professional role

  3. Survival strategies

    a. Inquire about being exempted from nursing courses through American College Testing Proficiency Examination Program—ACT PEP examinations (See Appendix A, ACT PEP Nursing Examination Chart, for more information)

    b. Inquire about obtaining academic credit for work experience

    c. Become familiar with course prerequisites, scheduling, and sequencing and with credit requirements to assist with planning

    d. Get to know academic advisor and maintain contact throughout the program to assist with problems and adjustment

    e. Allow extra time for studying

    f. Avoid using knowledge or experience to intimidate other students; treat them as peers

    g. Improve study and note-taking skills

    h. Avoid clinging to old ideas that may impede learning and professional growth

    i. Clarify and evaluate work and school values; retain important values and change or abandon others

    j. Keep an open mind and positive attitude toward instructors and classmates

    k. Share expertise and knowledge with instructors and classmates in a positive manner

    l. Seek advice from instructors when questions or concerns arise

    m. Keep career goals in mind as motivation for learning

E. RN entering college
1. Student characteristics
   a. Can be any age
   b. Experience in nursing care
   c. Motivation to enhance career credentials
   d. Committment to professional nursing
   e. Familiarity with aspects of the nursing curriculum
   f. Possible family and employment responsibilities
2. Problems encountered in adjusting to college
   a. Possible need to repeat nursing courses
   b. Conflict between work values and school values
   c. Unfamiliarity with course prerequisites, scheduling, and sequencing and with credit requirements
   d. Time management
   e. Feelings of superiority to instructor or classmates because of knowledge and work experience
   f. Role conflict between responsibilities as a student and those as an RN
3. Survival strategies
   a. Inquire about being exempted from nursing courses by taking ACT PEP examinations (see Appendix A for more information)
   b. Inquire about academic credit for work experience
   c. Become familiar with course prerequisites, sequencing, and scheduling and with credit requirements to assist with planning
   d. Get to know academic advisor and maintain contact throughout the program to help with adjustment and problems
   e. Allow extra time for studying
   f. Improve study and note-taking skills
   g. Avoid using knowledge and experience to intimidate other students; treat them as peers
   h. Avoid clinging to old ideas that impede learning and professional growth

i. Clarify and evaluate work values and school values; retain important values and change or abandon others
j. Keep an open mind and positive attitude toward instructors and classmates
k. Share expertise and knowledge with instructors and classmates in a positive manner
l. Seek advice from instructors when questions or concerns arise
m. Keep career goals in mind as motivation for learning
n. Know limits and responsibilities of a student to minimize role conflict

Points to Remember

Three basic education programs can lead to a nursing career: diploma, AD, and BSN.

Recent high school graduates entering college or nursing school and students who have been away from school for several years may find the adjustment difficult.

Nurses returning to college for academic degrees may experience conflict between the established professional role and the new student role.

Students returning to school after many years can ease the adjustment by reviewing study skills, planning for changes in family and work roles, and developing self-confidence.

All students entering college or nursing school can take steps to accommodate immediate life-style changes and eventual adjustment to a professional role.

Glossary

Academic advisor — professor or instructor assigned to provide guidance to individual students; assists with course selection, answers questions, and counsels students with academic problems

American College Testing Proficiency Examination Program (ACT PEP) — examinations for advanced placement in a nursing program; designed to help faculty and institutions establish credit-by-examination policies. Individual institutions establish standards for awarding credit

Credit — unit that measures amount of study a student must complete to qualify for an academic degree. For example, a course that meets for one semester hour per week carries one credit hour, one that meets for two semester hours per week carries two credit hours, and so forth. At least 60 credits are required for an AD; at least 120 credits are required for a BSN degree

Professional role — expectations and behaviors surrounding the practice of nursing influenced by nursing education, nurses in practice, professional associations, health care providers, and consumers, such as laypersons and patients

Role conflict — difficulties caused by taking on too many roles (professional or personal) simultaneously or having insufficient time to fulfill the responsibilities of all roles

Preparing for School

Learning Objectives
After studying this section, the reader should be able to:

- Discuss the importance of obtaining the support and cooperation of relatives and friends to achieve success in school.

- Describe strategies that can be used to obtain the support of others.

- Explain the importance of preparing for registration and learning details of the school's physical layout.

- Describe strategies to familiarize oneself with the logistics of registering for and attending school.

- Identify school services that assist students with academic or personal needs.

- Name student nurse organizations that address the concerns of nursing students.

II. Preparing for School

A. Introduction

1. A new school can be exciting and challenging, but it also can be confusing and frightening
2. Nursing school, regardless of its location in a community college, university, or hospital, can be overwhelming because of its size and complexity and the unfamiliarity of its surroundings
3. A prospective student can prepare for matriculation into a nursing program
4. Before classes begin:
   a. Obtain support from family or friends to minimize or avoid conflicts
   b. Become familiar with the layout of the school, hospital, and campus
   c. Prepare for registration to avoid errors in course selection
   d. Become familiar with the school's services
   e. Become familiar with student nursing organizations

B. Getting support

1. General information
   a. Support can be physical (for example, help with doing one's work) or emotional (for example, encouragement to continue working)
   b. Support systems can be formal or informal
   c. *Informal* support systems include family, friends, and other students
   d. Informal support systems provide comfort and sympathy; they do not necessarily require or effect change
   e. *Formal* support systems include organized, goal-oriented groups that require active member involvement
   f. In formal support systems, feelings and thoughts are shared and feedback is given to effect change
   g. Cooperation and support of family and friends can make success in school more probable
   h. Cooperation of employer and coworkers also is important
   i. The amount of support required depends on personal traits and circumstances
2. Survival strategies
   a. Discuss goals, time commitments, and demands of nursing school to gain understanding and maintain open communication with spouse or partner
   b. Involve spouse or partner in planning and decision making
   c. Reassure spouse or partner that commitment to school will not jeopardize the relationship with spouse or partner
   d. Discuss daily routines such as cooking, laundry, household chores, and children's extracurricular commitments to identify potential problems
   e. Tell children why school is important and how it will affect the family's schedule

    f. Reassure children that changes in the normal routine will not jeopardize their security

    g. Discuss school plans with employer to gain support and understanding

    h. Enlist employer's cooperation in planning work schedule to prevent conflicts with school schedule

    i. Reassure employer that job performance will not change

    j. Share plans with close colleagues to gain their support

    k. Identify colleagues willing to trade shifts or days off

    l. Be sensitive to colleagues' feelings; some may feel threatened

    m. Discuss school plans with friends; explain that although school will limit time for social activities, their friendship is still important

C. Logistics
1. General information
   a. A nursing school may be part of a large, sprawling campus or confined to a few buildings
   b. Typically, a nursing school at a community college or university is housed in one building with the other buildings for other courses such as business, engineering, and the sciences; the clinical affiliations usually are located in the neighboring area but are distinct and separate from the school
   c. A hospital-based nursing school can be housed in the hospital or in a separate building that is close to the hospital.
   d. At first glance, a school with many buildings and people can be overwhelming
   e. Nursing school and its clinical affiliations may be reached by public transportation or may require a car
   f. Familiarity with the layout of campus and buildings, and with means of access, can alleviate fear of getting lost and being late for class
2. Survival strategies
   a. Use a campus directory or map to learn layout and directions
   b. Find the buildings where classes are held before school starts to avoid delays
   c. Locate the department of nursing education
   d. Locate the offices of financial aid and of the bursar
   e. Locate the library, bookstore, cafeteria, and photocopying services
   f. Investigate public transportation
   g. Investigate the best route for driving; do a trial commute to estimate travel time
   h. Plan extra time for rush-hour commuting
   i. Locate student parking facilities and obtain parking sticker if necessary
   j. Locate clinical affiliations; investigate public transportation to these sites
   k. Inquire about parking facilities and fees at clinical sites

D. Registration
1. General information
   a. Registration is official enrollment in courses
   b. Registration usually occurs during the first few days of a semester
   c. All courses offered in a semester, along with day, time, and location of class, and credit hours given, are listed in a catalog or brochure
   d. Students choose classes according to the school they are enrolled in and their program requirements
   e. Students enrolled in diploma programs affiliated with a local college may have to register at the nursinc school *and* at the local college
   f. Students schedule classes according to personal needs and the availability of courses
   g. Registration can be overwhelming because of the many decisions that must be made
2. Survival strategies
   a. Know course requirements and course sequence before registration
   b. Discuss course selection with an academic advisor to help with program planning
   c. Decide which and how many courses to take each semester to fulfill credit and program requirements
   d. Be prepared to pay tuition or show evidence of waiver from the financial aid office; students cannot register without payment
   e. Register early on the first day to avoid finding courses filled
   f. Check the bookstore for required texts for each course
   g. Buy textbooks and supplies as soon as possible; inventory may be limited

E. School services
1. General information
   a. School services can help students cope with stress
   b. Available services are listed in the student manual
   c. An academic advisor may suggest special services to meet specific needs
   d. Services may include a learning resource center, counseling center, health center, and athletic facilities
2. Survival strategies
   a. Check the student manual for a list of student services
   b. Ask the academic advisor for help deciding which services would be useful
   c. Visit the learning resource center for help with reading, math, study, and writing skills
   d. Visit the counseling center for help with program planning, adjustment and personal problems, and career planning
   e. Visit the health center for care of minor illnesses, reproductive health care services, psychological services, and assistance for handicapped students
   f. Investigate athletic facilities for fitness and sports programs

F. Student nurse organizations
1. General information
   a. A school student nurse organization may address issues of concern within the school as well as on the local, state, and national levels
   b. All states have a student nurse organization that operates with the support of the state nurses' association to involve students in state issues
   c. Student nurse organizations sponsor workshops and conventions
   d. Students can join state or national student nurse associations even if their own school does not have a student nurse organization
   e. The National Student Nurses' Association (NSNA) is the organization for students in nursing school
   f. The NSNA is an independent organization that works closely with the American Nurses' Association (ANA)
   g. NSNA members serve on ANA committees; they provide a student viewpoint on issues
   h. The NSNA developed a Student Bill of Rights that outlines the rights and responsibilities of students
   i. The Student Bill of Rights deals with the education program, the rules and policies of the institution, and freedom in personal decision making
2. Survival strategies
   a. Join a school organization and become active in its work to meet classmates and learn about issues of concern
   b. Join the state student nurse association to meet student nurses from other schools and to learn about state-level issues (see Appendix B, Professional Nursing Organizations Directory, for a list of professional organizations)
   c. Join NSNA to learn about national issues
   d. Participate in the organization's activities

Points to Remember

The support and cooperation of spouse, children, employer, coworkers, and friends are vital to achieving success in school.

Familiarity with school logistics will reduce anxiety and stress.

Registration is official enrollment in courses for a semester. It requires familiarity with program requirements, credits, and course sequencing.

School services can help meet the academic, health care, emotional, and physical needs of students.

The NSNA is the organization for students in nursing school.

Glossary

Clinical affiliation — agency separate from the school or college used for clinical experience; usually a hospital, nursing home, or community health agency

National Student Nurses' Association (NSNA) — organization for nursing school students

School services — programs designed to assist students with special needs by providing academic assistance, counseling, health care, or athletic facilities

Student manual — book published by the school describing all aspects of student life

Financial Assistance

Learning Objectives

After studying this section, the reader should be able to:

- Discuss the most common types of financial assistance available to college students.

- Describe how a needs analysis is used to determine eligibility for financial assistance.

- Describe the process of applying for financial assistance and the importance of filing applications early.

- Describe the role of the financial aid officer.

III. Financial Assistance

A. Introduction

1. Nursing education can be expensive, but financial assistance is available
2. The student must know how, when, and where to apply to receive financial assistance
3. Sources of financial assistance include the federal and state governments, educational institutions, private institutions, and employer-sponsored programs
4. Financial assistance may be grants or scholarships, which need not be repaid, or loans, which must be repaid
5. Employment arranged by the school's financial aid office also provides financial assistance
6. An applicant must meet eligibility requirements to receive financial assistance
7. Factors that determine eligibility include enrollment status, school accreditation, and student status
8. Some federal and state aid packages require that a student be enrolled for a minimum of half-time study
   a. Half-time study is defined differently by schools using semester hours, credit hours, clock hours, or trimester and quarter systems
   b. Proof of satisfactory academic progress may be required to maintain eligibility after the first year
9. An institution must be nationally accredited for students to qualify for federal or state aid
10. Financial assistance programs define students as dependent or independent
    a. *Dependent* students rely at least partially on their parents for financial support
    b. *Independent* students do not rely on parents for financial support
11. Federal regulations state that a student classified as *independent* must fit one of the following categories
    a. Be age 24 by December 31 of the award year
    b. Be an orphan, ward of the court, or veteran of the Armed Services
    c. Have legal dependents other than a spouse
    d. Be married, a professional student, or a graduate student, and not be claimed as a dependent for tax purposes by a parent for the first year of the award year
    e. Be a single undergraduate, under age 24, with no dependents, and not be claimed as a dependent for tax purposes by a parent for either of the two calendar years preceding the award year; demonstrate self-sufficiency by showing an income of at least $4000 in each of those two years
    f. Be judged independent by the financial aid officer (FAO), based on documented circumstances

B. Institutional loans
1. Before an institution considers a request for financial assistance, it determines how much the applicant can afford to pay; this is called *needs analysis*
   a. Needs analysis is performed by the College Board's College Scholarship Service or the American College Testing Program
   b. Both services review the student's (or family's) finances, and apply a standard formula to determine how much the student can be expected to pay
2. If the amount is less than the cost of attending the institution of choice, the student is determined to have financial need
3. The FAO plays a major role in determining eligibility for and amount of financial assistance
   a. The FAO can increase or decrease the amount of family contribution identified by the needs analysis
   b. The FAO can allocate money controlled by the institution or certify the student's eligibility for money from other sources
   c. The FAO determines the percentage of loans, grants, and scholarships that make up the total financial assistance package

C. Student loans
1. Federal loans
   a. The federal government offers low-interest loans to assist students with college expenses
   b. Interest on some loans is paid by the government while the student is enrolled in school
   c. The government may guarantee the loan against default
   d. The loan may be deferred or cancelled in exchange for public service work, such as a 2-year commitment to the Indian Health Service
   e. A 6- to 9-month grace period after graduation may be granted before repayment of the loan begins
2. Stafford Loans (formerly Guaranteed Student Loans)
   a. Low-interest loans for undergraduate and graduate students who are U.S. citizens or resident aliens and who are enrolled at least half-time
   b. Loan limits are up to $2,625 per year for freshmen and sophomores; up to $4,000 per year for juniors, seniors, and fifth-year undergraduates
   c. Maximum loan for undergraduate education is $17,250
   d. Lenders are banks, savings and loan associations, insurance companies, and credit unions
   e. Interest rate is 8% for the first 4 years of repayment, and 10% thereafter
   f. Lenders may charge an insurance fee of up to 3% of the amount of the outstanding loan
   g. Students attending accredited colleges, universities, and nursing and vocational schools are eligible

     h. Applicants must show "remaining need" — the difference between the cost of attending school and the student's contribution plus scholarships, grants, and other benefits

     i. Repayment begins after graduation

3. Parent Loans to Undergraduate Students (PLUS)-Supplemental Loans to Students (SLS)

     a. Loan limits are up to $4,000 per year to a maximum of $20,000

     b. Parents may have to pass a credit check when applying for PLUS

     c. SLS loans are restricted to professional students, graduate students, and independent undergraduate students

     d. SLS applicants must attend school at least half-time and must apply for Stafford Loan and Pell Grant (see page 26) before being considered for SLS

     e. Lenders are banks, savings and loan associations, credit unions, and insurance companies

     f. Interest rate is adjusted annually, with a 12% maximum; interest accrues during all periods of the loan, including deferments

     g. Repayment of principal and interest begins within 60 days after the loan is taken out

4. Carl D. Perkins loans

     a. Loans are administered by colleges for undergraduate and graduate students with demonstrated need

     b. Loan funds are allocated to schools by the federal government

     c. Loan limits are $4,500 for a vocational program or the first two years of a baccalaureate program; $9,000 for third-year students; $18,000 for graduate students

     d. Interest rate is 5%; student does not pay interest while attending school, during deferments, or during the 6-month grace period that follows each deferment

     e. Generous deferment policies apply for Peace Corps, Volunteers in Service to America, and other public service work, as well as for students in internships or on parental leave, and working mothers

     f. Loans are repaid by the federal government in exchange for service in the National Guard or military reserve, and for active military duty

     g. A 9-month grace period after graduation is granted before repayment begins

     h. Perkins loans are not equally available at all schools; the amount allotted a school depends on its student default rate for repayment

5. Nursing student loans

     a. Loans are given to half-time and full-time students at schools of professional nursing

     b. Accredited public and nonprofit private schools of nursing are eligible

     c. Loan funds from banks and nursing organizations are allocated to schools, which select the recipients

     d. Loan limits are $2,500 per year to a total of $10,000

e. Interest rate is 6%; student does not pay interest while in school or during deferments

f. Deferments are given for full-time graduate study, and for military service and service in the U.S. Public Health Department or the Peace Corps

g. Repayment begins 9 months after completing studies (or deferment) and extends over ten years

h. Program operates on revolving funds: Schools must collect payment on outstanding loans to have money for new loans

i. At present, 80% of nursing schools are in danger of having funds cut because of high default rate

6. Pell Grants

a. Cash awards for undergraduate students enrolled at least half-time; need not be repaid

b. 7,000 colleges, universities, vocational schools, and accredited hospital schools of nursing are eligible

c. Rules and regulations change frequently; application is complicated and time-consuming

d. Eligibility is based on a formula applied to personal financial information submitted with the application and resulting in a Pell Grant Index (PGI)

e. PGI ranges from 0 to 2,100; 0 qualifies for maximum assistance, 2,100 for minimum assistance; student with index greater than 2,100 is ineligible

f. At present, maximum award is $2,300; amount changes regularly

g. Notification of eligibility usually not received until after the student has been accepted by a college

h. Lack of federal appropriations or problems with the federal budget can leave less money for Pell Grants, making award smaller than originally anticipated

i. Most colleges require students to apply for a Pell Grant before considering them for a Stafford Student Loan or SLS Loan

j. Application should be made immediately after January 1 to allow as much time as possible to apply for other aid

7. Supplemental Educational Opportunity Grants (SEOGs)

a. SEOGs are federal grants for full- or half-time undergraduates with exceptional financial need; they need not be repaid

b. Each school participating in the program receives a certain amount of money; when that money is gone, no further grants can be made

c. Award amount depends on the recipient's resources and the availability of funds at the school

8. College Work Study (CWS)

a. Provides jobs for undergraduate and graduate students who need financial assistance

b. Federal funds are made available to participating schools and colleges; jobs are awarded as part of financial assistance packages

c. The student receives money from the fund in addition to the wages from the job

d. Pay is at least current federal minimum wage; undergraduates are paid by the hour, graduate students may be salaried

e. Jobs are usually on campus, working for the school (in the cafeteria or library, for example); or off campus, with a nonprofit organization or state or federal agency

f. Work schedule is set by the school

9. Junior fellowships

a. This federally-sponsored program for students in top 10% of high school class who demonstrate financial need

b. The program provides opportunities for students to work in federal agencies during academic breaks

c. Application and selection of recipients are made in senior year of high school

d. Fellowship limit is up to $12,500 over four years

e. Fellowships usually result in employment after graduation

f. Lack of publicity has kept program underused; therefore fellowships are usually available

10. State programs

a. State aid programs include grants, tuition assistance, fee reductions, and loans

b. States have reciprocal agreements that allow students from one state to attend college in another state at reduced tuition

c. Certain loan programs waive loan repayment for students willing to study teaching, medicine, nursing, education, or other fields in which the state is experiencing shortages

d. Special programs exist for minority students, veterans, National Guard members, and military dependents

e. Some states are developing prepaid tuition plans that enable parents to guarantee four years at a state college

f. Many states give merit awards for academic achievement; these are unrelated to financial need

g. Many states administer work-study programs similar to federal programs

11. Private programs

a. Many private institutions offer financial aid from private sources

b. Private funds may be paid in addition to state and federal assistance

c. All education institutions have endowments for scholarship aid and make these awards independently; they are awarded for academic excellence and are not based on financial need

d. Some schools offer more scholarship choices after a student successfully completes the freshman year

e. Corporations may establish scholarships for children of employees and retirees

f. Civic and fraternal organizations may offer scholarships for local students

g. Private foundation funds are available, usually to graduate and doctoral students

h. Organizations such as the Nurses Educational Funds (NEF) offer scholarships for graduate nursing education, ranging from $2,500 to $6,000

12. Tuition aid from employers
    a. Many hospitals, nursing homes, and corporations offer full or partial tuition reimbursement for employees
    b. Reimbursement may be a free benefit, or may require repayment in the form of employment at the institution for a specified number of years
    c. Most tuition reimbursement programs require that courses be job-related
    d. Many employers require a specified length of employment before eligibility for reimbursement begins
13. Cooperative education
    a. Cooperative education combines academic study with a related off-campus job; program length is usually 5 years
    b. In most cases, money earned covers tuition cost
    c. Under the *alternating method*, the student studies full-time for a semester or term, then works full-time for the next semester or term; the cycle repeats until graduation
    d. Under the *parallel method*, the student attends classes part-time and works part-time
    e. Under the *extended day method*, the student works full-time and attends evening classes

D. **Application for financial assistance**
   1. General information
      a. Financial planning requires knowledge of the sources of financial assistance, and application procedures and deadlines
      b. The public library, high school guidance counselors, and college financial aid offices are good sources of information on financial assistance (see *Financial resource information* for additional sources)
      c. Federal and state regulations related to loans and grants change frequently
   2. Survival strategies
      a. Obtain a reasonably comprehensive, *current* book on financial assistance
      b. Use college catalogs to learn about financial assistance offered by the school; ask an advisor or FAO about details
      c. Present financial need as strongly as legally possible for the needs analysis
      d. Investigate student loans available through banks and savings and loan societies
      e. Apply to all major assistance programs
      f. Apply for assistance *early*, and complete forms *thoroughly*, to avoid delays in processing
      g. Apply for a Stafford or PLUS-SLS loan by locating the lender and sending an application to the college of choice; college certifies information and returns it to lender; lender submits form to guaranteeing agency; agency issues promissory note; applicant signs promissory note and returns it to lender

h. Get to know the institution's FAO, who can influence the composition of students' assistance packages

i. Check with the financial aid office annually about scholarships or grants available only to students who have completed a year of study

j. When job hunting after graduation, look for employers who offer tuition reimbursement

k. If already employed, investigate employer's tuition reimbursement program; understand eligibility terms and any commitments required

l. If lack of money threatens continued study, discuss the situation with the FAO; emergency assistance is commonly available to help meet extraordinary needs

m. If financial assistance is contingent on "satisfactory academic achievement," begin with a light course load to avoid risking loss of assistance

FINANCIAL RESOURCE INFORMATION

The following organizations are useful sources of information about financial assistance.

American Association of Colleges of Nursing
One Dupont Circle NW Suite 530
Washington, D.C. 20036
(202) 463-6930

Federal Student Aid Information
(800) 333-INFO
For information about program requirements, eligibility verification, filing applications, or explanations of the awards process, call Monday-Friday 9:00 a.m.-5:30 p.m.

National Commission for Cooperative Education
360 Huntington Avenue
Boston, MA 02115
(617) 437-3778
For free information on undergraduate and graduate cooperative education

National League for Nursing
10 Columbus Circle
New York, NY 10019
(212) 582-1022

National Student Nurses Association
555 West 57th Street, #1325
New York, NY 10019
(212) 581-2211

Nurses Educational Funds
555 West 57th Street, 13th Floor
New York, NY 10019
(212) 582-8820
For information about NEF scholarships for graduate nursing education

Nursing Student Loans
Division of Student Assistance, Room 8-44
5600 Fishers Lane
Rockville, MD 20857
(301) 443-1173

Octameron Associates
P.O. Box 3437, Alexandria, VA 22302
Don't Miss Out: The Ambitious Student's Guide to Financial Aid 1989-90, 13th ed. ($5.00) By Robert Leider and Anna Leider.

Book covering loans, grants, scholarships, and financial management techniques for undergraduate and graduate education

Project on Status of Education and Women
Association of American Colleges
1818 R Street, NW
Washington, D.C. 20009
(202) 387-1300

Points to Remember

Financial assistance for students is available from the federal and state governments and from private sources.

The institution's FAO has final responsibility for the financial assistance package offered to a student.

Most financial aid packages include several types of assistance, including low-interest loans, scholarships, grants, and work-study programs.

The student should gather information on all types of financial assistance, complete the application accurately, and meet application deadlines.

Glossary

Enrollment status — the number of hours a student is enrolled in the institution; full-time, half-time, or part-time (usually less than half-time)

Grant — cash award that need not be repaid

Loan — money borrowed from a bank or savings and loan society; must be repaid

Student status — academic standing; typically one of the criteria necessary to qualify for or retain financial assistance

Work-study program — employment arranged by an institution to help a student meet school-related expenses; considered financial assistance

The Curriculum

Learning Objectives

After studying this section, the reader should be able to:

- Define a nursing program curriculum.

- Identify the factors that shape a curriculum.

- Explain the importance of learning objectives.

- Describe the purpose of the course outline and its significance to students.

- Discuss the faculty and its significance to students.

...culum is the study plan for an educational program

...rsing programs have certain requirements, known as prerequisites, for ...mission into the program; common prerequisites include a high school diploma or equivalency, 2 years of mathematics, a chemistry course, and a biology course

3. The nursing curriculum includes courses that provide a student with the knowledge and skills necessary to become a nurse

4. The nursing curriculum is based on a philosophy, a conceptual framework, and learning objectives (see *Curriculum plan*)

5. Organization and sequence of nursing courses vary with nursing programs
   a. In diploma and associate degree nursing programs, nursing courses begin immediately; the student takes science courses concurrently
   b. In baccalaureate degree nursing programs, nursing courses begin late in the second year or in the third year of the program; the student takes liberal arts and science courses for the first two years

6. The nursing program curriculum is listed in the school catalog and is discussed during the orientation program

7. The orientation program:
   a. Provides an overview of the curriculum, including philosophy, conceptual framework, and learning objectives
   b. Briefly explains course content, prerequisites, and sequence
   c. Identifies attendance requirements for classes, laboratories, and clinical learning activities
   d. Provides an overview of course grading policies; for example, the number of examinations and the method for determining final grades
   e. Explains the evaluation procedure for clinical learning; for example, a letter grade or pass-fail system
   f. Explains promotion policy; for example, grade point average (GPA) needed to continue in the nursing program
   g. Explains dismissal policy; for example, the consequences of unsatisfactory clinical evaluation, excessive absence, or failure to achieve minimum GPA

8. Survival strategies
   a. Organize written copies of program policies, procedures, and course requirements in a notebook for reference
   b. Ask about policies and procedures
   c. Refer to written policy when student status is an issue
   d. Review policies, procedures, and course requirements periodically

B. Philosophy
1. General information
   a. Offers a statement of the program faculty's beliefs and values about nursing and nursing education, consistent with the philosophy of the parent institution

CURRICULUM PLAN

Each school's philosophy provides the foundation for its curriculum. The concepts, ideas, and values identified in the philosophy are embodied in each aspect of the curriculum.

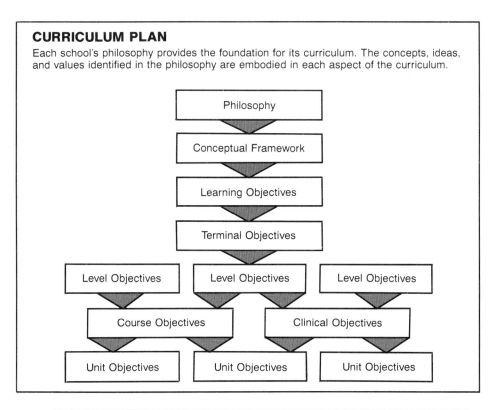

   b. Defines curriculum structure, which directly relates to nursing course content and sequencing and to clinical activities

   c. Reflects values of the philosophy in course content and clinical learning requirements

2. Survival strategies

   a. Identify personal values and beliefs about nursing and nursing education and be certain that they correspond to the values and beliefs of the nursing program

   b. Be aware that the values and beliefs stated in the philosophy will be reflected in each course and commonly are the areas on which students are tested

   c. Plan to integrate values and beliefs into clinical and classroom work

C. Conceptual framework

1. General information

   a. Offers a model or blueprint for the nursing curriculum that provides a picture of the curriculum as a whole rather than as a collection of individual courses

       b. Identifies the focus or concept—such as nursing process, health, and adaptation—that is common to all nursing courses
       c. Establishes logical course sequencing and consistency throughout courses
       d. Guides faculty in selecting appropriate clinical learning activities

  2. Survival strategies
       a. Use the conceptual framework as a guide for applying theoretical knowledge to nursing care
       b. Focus learning on the concepts identified by the conceptual framework; these concepts often provide a basis for examination
       c. Use the conceptual framework to provide a unified picture of the curriculum as a whole rather than as a collection of individual courses

D. Objectives
  1. General information
       a. Objectives provide goals to be achieved
       b. Objectives are stated in behavioral terms
       c. *Learning* objectives are specific, measurable goals for acquiring knowledge, including course objectives, clinical objectives, level objectives, and terminal objectives (see *Examples of learning objectives*)
       d. *Course* objectives describe behaviors a student should demonstrate upon completion of a course; they can be divided into unit objectives and lecture objectives

EXAMPLES OF LEARNING OBJECTIVES

Learning objectives provide specific goals and serve as guides for study. Here are some examples:

Course Objective
At the conclusion of the course, the student will use theoretical knowledge of pathophysiology to facilitate adaptive behavior in patients with changes in oxygen utilization.

Level Objectives
At the conclusion of Level 2, the student will:
- interpret data and identify nursing diagnosis
- assist clients in setting goals and making decisions about health care
- organize nursing actions to meet the needs of one or two patients.

Unit Objectives
At the conclusion of the unit, the student will:
- describe subjective and objective data for a respiratory assessment
- describe signs and symptoms commonly associated with respiratory disorders
- identify the major defining characteristics and expected outcomes of the following nursing diagnosis: Ineffective Airway Clearance.

Clinical Objective
During clinical learning experience, the student will perform a respiratory assessment of an assigned patient.

    e. *Clinical* objectives describe behaviors a student should demonstrate during a clinical learning experience

    f. *Level* objectives describe behaviors a student should demonstrate at the completion of each level or year of study

    g. *Terminal* objectives describe behaviors a student should demonstrate at the completion of the program

2. Survival strategies

    a. Keep in mind that course objections identify the most important course content, so review objectives periodically to refocus attention on important areas

    b. Use course, clinical, and level objections to plan for study, course assignments, examinations, and clinical learning activities, and for self-assessment at the end of each course or semester

    c. Review course, clinical, and level objectives to evaluate performance and make adjustments for improvement as necessary

    d. Use terminal objectives for self-assessment at the completion of the program and as a review guide

    e. Review clinical objectives before clinical experience because the clinical instructor will use these objectives to evaluate student performance

E. Course outline

1. General information

    a. Describes theoretical content and scope of instruction in the course

    b. Identifies course prerequisites and placement in the curriculum

    c. Lists learning objectives

    d. Provides course hours for lectures, laboratories, and clinical activities

    e. Identifies teaching methods used, such as lecture, demonstration, audiovisuals, clinical practice

    f. Identifies requirements for assignments, and explains testing and grading

    g. Defines attendance policy

    h. Lists required textbooks

    i. Identifies evaluation methods

    j. May include additional reading assignments from nursing journals and other sources

    k. May provide a syllabus (a calendar of classes, including which topics will be covered during each class)

2. Survival strategies

    a. Use the course outline as a guide for reading and studying

    b. Use the outline to know the requirements for attendance, assignments, testing, and grading

    c. Ask the instructor to clarify requirements

    d. Buy textbooks early; bookstore's inventory may be limited

    e. Gather required articles early

    f. Use the syllabus to prepare for classes and plan ahead for assignments, review, and study

F. Faculty

1. General information
   a. Instructors vary in classroom approach, teaching style, personality, educational preparation, and title
   b. Instructors' educational preparation varies according to the institution and type of nursing program
   c. National League for Nursing (NLN) requires a master's degree for theoretical teaching in an accredited nursing program
   d. NLN requires a bachelor's degree for clinical teaching in an accredited nursing program
   e. Faculty titles are based on criteria established by the institution
   f. *Adjunct faculty* are part-time employees, usually responsible for teaching one course
   g. *Nursing instructors* may have a bachelor's or master's degree, with clinical expertise in one or more areas of nursing; they may be full-time or part-time faculty
   h. *Assistant professors* may have a master's degree or doctorate; they usually hold a full-time position and have spent a required number of years at the institution
   i. *Professors* have a doctorate degree and full-time academic responsibility, have spent a required number of years at the institution, and have tenure
   j. *Dean*, *associate dean*, and *division chairperson* are titles accorded to individuals with administrative responsibility and authority within an institution; academic administrators usually have a doctorate
2. Survival strategies
   a. Get to know instructors personally to improve communication
   b. Avoid judging instructors too soon; first impressions may be incorrect
   c. Discuss problems directly with instructors to avoid confusion
   d. Do not let personality conflicts with instructors interfere with learning
   e. Adapt to the instructor's style to get the most out of a course
   f. Do not argue with instructors; it interferes with learning
   g. Learn everything possible from a course, whether or not an instructor meets your expectations
   h. Address an instructor by academic title to show courtesy and respect
   i. When in doubt about a title, use Mr., Mrs., or Ms. with the person's surname
   j. Do not use an instructor's first name unless requested to do so

Points to Remember

The nursing curriculum is developed from an institution's philosophy and conceptual framework; it will vary among programs and schools.

Orientation to the nursing program provides an overview of the program and a description of courses, requirements, and policies.

Learning objectives identify specific goals for learning and provide a focus for studying.

A course outline describes the theoretical content and scope of instruction in the course.

Instructors vary in educational preparation, title, classroom approach, style, and personality.

Glossary

Conceptual framework — model for the curriculum based on nursing theory or other concepts

Curriculum — body of courses offered to teach theoretical knowledge and clinical skills

Philosophy — statement of faculty beliefs about nursing and nursing education

Syllabus — document listing information about a course, such as lecture topics, readings, assignments, and bibliography

Tenure — instructor's status achieved by meeting an institution's requirements for advanced education, publication, and years of service

Classroom Skills

Learning Objectives

After studying this section, the reader should be able to:

● Describe the kinds of classes that make up a nursing program.

● Explain the importance of preparing for class, and describe strategies for successful preparation.

● Explain the importance of listening skills, and describe strategies for improving them.

● Explain the importance of note-taking skills, and describe strategies for successful note-taking.

V. Classroom Skills

A. Introduction

1. A student can improve classroom learning by developing techniques to enhance memory and retention
2. Techniques can improve learning
   a. Recognize individual learning style
   b. Prepare for class
   c. Sharpen listening skills
   d. Improve note-taking skills
3. Techniques used are influenced by type of class being taken
   a. Type of class depends on the subject being taught, number of students in the class, space available, and institutional resources
   b. Nursing students attend lectures, seminars and discussion groups, and laboratory classes
   c. Every type of class may not suit every student's individual learning style
   d. Regardless of type of class, student should be prepared to listen and take notes
   e. Regardless of individual learning style, student must prepare to learn
4. A *lecture* is the most common type of class in a college or nursing school
   a. A lecture may be attended by numerous students, ranging from 30 to 200
   b. In a lecture, the instructor speaks from prepared notes and may use slides, an overhead projector, or other visual aids
   c. Lectures may include an opportunity to ask questions, but limited opportunity for class discussion
5. Seminars and discussion groups also are part of the nursing curriculum
   a. A *seminar* usually consists of 10 to 20 students
   b. A seminar provides an opportunity to ask questions, share thoughts, and discuss ideas
6. A *laboratory class* may be part of a science course, such as Anatomy and Physiology, or a nursing course, such as Nursing Fundamentals
   a. A laboratory class usually consists of 10 to 20 students
   b. A teaching assistant or a professor may teach the theory component of the course
   c. A laboratory class provides an opportunity for practical learning, such as scientific demonstration, experimentation, or practice of clinical procedures
7. Survival strategies
   a. Become familiar with the structure of individual classes
   b. Try to accommodate your individual learning style to the classroom situation
   c. Come to class prepared to be an active learner

   d. Be aware of personal learning style; determine whether best results are achieved by reading, listening, seeing pictures, writing, or asking questions
   e. If reading is most helpful, read as much relevant material as possible (in addition to what is assigned) before class
   f. If seeing pictures is most helpful, sit up front to see visual aids
   g. If listening is most helpful, sit up front to hear better
   h. If repetition is most helpful, tape the lecture for later listening
   i. If writing is most helpful, take careful notes; when studying from texts, paraphrase material in simple language
   j. If asking questions is most helpful, be prepared to participate in class

B. Class preparation
   1. General information
      a. Preparation consists of reading textbook chapters and completing other assignments *before* attending class
      b. Amount and type of class preparation varies according to the course content and the instructor's requirements
      c. Preparation enhances learning because the student is not encountering information for the first time in class
      d. Familiarity with a topic helps the student understand the instructor, take notes, and ask questions
      e. Preparation for class demonstrates interest in the course
   2. Survival strategies
      a. Use the course outline or syllabus to identify material that will be covered in class
      b. Refer to the course outline or syllabus to identify related readings
      c. Read for an overview of the topic
      d. Prepare questions that clarify difficult or confusing concepts or statements
      e. Review textbook diagrams and graphics to increase your familiarity with the topic
      f. Look up and jot down definitions of unfamiliar words

C. Listening Skills
   1. General information
      a. Much learning can occur through listening
      b. Hearing is a selective process; an individual can listen actively for every detail or can block out unwanted or extraneous information or noise
      c. Barriers to comprehensive listening include a negative attitude, lack of interest, dislike of the instructor's personality or mannerisms, and inability to concentrate
      d. Different types of classes may require different listening skills
      e. Listening skills can be practiced and refined (see *Listening skills*)

2. Survival strategies: Lectures
   a. Sit up front to improve vision and hearing
   b. Look directly at the lecturer to improve concentration
   c. Ignore distractions inside or outside the room
   d. Focus on the lecture; do not daydream or doodle
   e. Listen for key phrases, such as *The four major theories are...; The important point is...; The implications for nursing care are...*
   f. Note the kinds of questions the lecturer asks; for example, do the questions relate theory to clinical situations or do they investigate pathophysiology?
   g. Note if the lecturer covers textbook material or introduces material not contained in the text
   h. Take advantage of such visual aids as charts, diagrams, and graphs
   i. Ask *Why is this important?* to help focus on practical applications
3. Survival strategies: Seminars or group discussions
   a. Listen actively to others; avoid formulating a response while someone else is speaking
   b. Remember that everyone has personal values and beliefs; avoid arguing about them
   c. Respond to others' viewpoints; avoid making speeches
   d. Do not make insulting or demeaning comments; this inflames others and weakens legitimate points
   e. Do not monopolize discussions; this interferes with other students' learning
4. Survival strategies: Laboratory classes
   a. Listen actively to directions for experiments or procedures
   b. Concentrate on the instructor's demonstrations
   c. Use such visual aids as charts, diagrams, and models to help reinforce demonstrations
   d. Ask *Why is this important?*

LISTENING SKILLS

AIDS TO LISTENING	BLOCKS TO LISTENING
● Sit in the front of the room ● Ignore distractions ● Listen for key words: The *most important* concept is... The *four major* categories are... The *most common* signs and symptoms are... ● Develop an interest in the topic	● Mind wandering to other subjects ● Daydreaming ● Doodling or drawing ● Lack of interest, boredom

D. Note-taking skills
1. General information
   a. Class notes should summarize a lecture, seminar, or discussion
   b. Laboratory class notes should record observations or provide details of an experiment or procedure
   c. Class notes should capture the most important points of a lecture; they should not be verbatim transcripts
   d. Class notes should include questions asked by the instructor, which are clues to what the instructor considers important
   e. Class notes should include examples or sketches used by the instructor, which may help jog memory
   f. Tape-recorded lectures can be useful but should not replace class notes
   g. Class notes are essential for study and review
2. Survival strategies
   a. Keep all course notes in one notebook for easy reference
   b. Date all notes to identify lecture topic and time; include the instructor's name
   c. Allow adequate space for notes; cramming information into small spaces makes reading and review difficult
   d. Listen actively; write quickly to avoid missing information while writing
   e. Do not try to write every word spoken; listen for understanding and write key words and phrases only
   f. Use abbreviations and symbols such as = (equals), # (number), & (and), and gtt (drops), to save time
   g. Write legibly to avoid confusion later
   h. Draw pictures or diagrams to jog memory during review
   i. Obtain the instructor's permission before you tape a lecture
   j. Use tape recordings for particularly difficult classes or to fill in gaps in notes
   k. Do not rely solely on tape recording; note-taking helps focus attention and improves listening skills
   l. Review notes as soon as possible after a lecture to reinforce learning and improve memory
   m. Highlight or underline key points and new vocabulary
   n. Fill in gaps that occurred during class; rely on memory, consult classmates, or refer to a textbook for missing information
   o. Summarize information by paraphrasing the instructor's language, which can reinforce learning
   p. Write questions to ask at the next class

Points to Remember

Nursing students attend lectures, seminars and discussion groups, and laboratory classes.

Preparation for class facilitates learning.

Active listening skills are developed by concentrating on the instructor, listening for key words, and ignoring distractions.

Class notes should summarize the main points of a lecture.

Using abbreviations, pictures, and symbols saves time and facilitates note-taking.

Notes should be reviewed soon after class and regularly throughout the course to improve memory and facilitate learning.

Glossary

Laboratory — class in which students practice what they have learned in lectures and seminars; used in science courses and in nursing courses on clinical procedures, interviewing techniques, and physical assessment skills

Lecture — traditional college class format in which the instructor speaks from prepared notes

Seminar — class in which students are responsible for planning, presenting, and leading or participating in discussion according to the instructor's guidelines

Communication Skills

Learning Objectives

After studying this section, the reader should be able to:

- Define communication.

- Identify factors that influence communication.

- Explain the two primary methods of communication.

- Discuss survival strategies related to each method of communication.

VI. Communication Skills

A. Introduction

1. All people have a basic need to relate to others
2. Communication is a way to fulfill this need
3. Communication is dynamic and ongoing
   a. A way to interact and develop relationships
   b. A way to effect change
4. Communication involves transmitting messages from a sender to a receiver
   a. The *message* is a series of words that may be accompanied by gestures
   b. The *sender* transmits the message with a specific meaning
   c. The *receiver* of the message absorbs the information and may return a response (feedback) to the sender
5. The receiver can interpret a message in different ways, and not necessarily as the sender intended
6. Factors that affect how a receiver interprets a message include:
   a. Perceptions
   b. Values
   c. Emotions
   d. Sociocultural background
   e. Level of knowledge
   f. Role in relationship
   g. Setting
7. Communication is effective when the receiver interprets the message as the sender intended it
8. Techniques that promote effective communication include:
   a. Stating observations
   b. Restating
   c. Clarifying
   d. Offering information
   e. Using open-ended questions
   f. Paraphrasing
   g. Reflecting
   h. Focusing
   i. Listening attentively
   j. Validating
   k. Summarizing
9. Techniques that block communication include:
   a. Using close-ended questions
   b. Offering advice or opinions
   c. Making judgments
   d. Changing the subject
   e. Offering false reassurance
   f. Using cliches
   g. Being defensive

10. Communication forms the basis of relationships
    a. Relationships can be social or therapeutic
    b. A *social* relationship meets the needs of both people involved
    c. A *therapeutic* relationship meets the needs of the receiver, but not necessarily those of the sender
11. Nursing students have both kinds of relationships
    a. Social relationships involve classmates, colleagues, and friends
    b. Therapeutic relationships involve patients in a clinical setting
12. In both types of relationships, messages are sent and received

B. Verbal communication
1. General information
   a. Verbal communications is the transmission of messages using spoken or written language
   b. Language is affected by social, economic, and cultural background, age, and education
   c. Consequently, a message can mean one thing to the sender and another to the receiver
   d. Criteria to be considered when communicating verbally include simplicity, clarity, timing, relevance, adaptability, and credibility
   e. *Simplicity* refers to stating complex idea in commonly understood terms, using short sentences that express the idea completely
   f. *Clarity* refers to using words to state exactly what is meant so that the receiver need not make any assumptions
   g. *Timing* and *relevance* refer to ensuring that the message is communicated at a time when the receiver is ready to receive it and in an appropriate form
   h. *Adaptability* refers to stating the message in a way that reflects on the situation and shows appropriateness to the receiver
   i. *Credibility* refers to stating the message in a trustworthy and believable manner, being accurate and confident, consistent and honest
   j. For verbal communication to be effective, these criteria need to be met
   k. Throughout nursing school, students need to communicate with other students, instructors, friends, and patients: this communication occurs through the spoken and written word
   l. Students use the spoken word with friends, colleagues, instructors, and patients
   m. Students use the written word in documenting, preparing nursing care plans, and in presenting research reports
2. Survival strategies
   a. Assess verbal communication, including speaking and writing styles, and how messages are received; identify and improve problem areas

  b. State complex ideas in short sentences, using easily understood language; avoid unnecessary technical terms and jargon
  c. Use unambiguous words to avoid misinterpretation
  d. Speak at a reasonable rate for clarity, and enunciate clearly
  e. Avoid generalizing and expressing opinions
  f. Use appropriate timing
  g. Communicate accurately, confidently, and honestly
  h. Be sensitive to others' needs and feelings; personalize communication
  i. Do not be afraid to say "I don't know"; be aware of personal limitations and try to correct them
  j. Observe and evaluate how listeners respond to messages

C. Nonverbal communication
  1. General information
      a. Transmits messages without using words (commonly called *body language*)
      b. Includes hand gestures, body movements, physical appearance, posture, gait, and facial expressions
      c. Conveys feelings such as joy, sadness, anger, and anxiety rather than ideas
      d. Reflects self-concept, current mood, and health
      e. Helps interpret spoken messages
      f. Requires acute observation by the receiver for accurate interpretation of the message
      g. Used by student nurses with classmates, friends, instructors, and patients
      h. Helps in interactions with patients
  2. Survival strategies
      a. Assess personal style; ask others for assessments
      b. Practice before a mirror to identify positive and negative expressions and gestures
      c. Observe others' nonverbal communication styles
      d. Use all senses when listening to concentrate on the message being sent
      e. Face listeners when speaking to show interest and availability
      f. Maintain eye contact when speaking and listening
      g. Assume non defensive posture to encourage communication; do not cross arms or legs, which can imply impatience or lack of interest
      h. Maintain a neat appearance to invite communication

Points to Remember

Communication, a dynamic, ongoing process, provides a foundation for relationships and a means to effect change.

Communication involves a message, a sender, and a receiver.

Communication can be verbal, through written or spoken words, or nonverbal, through body language and appearance.

Nursing students use verbal and nonverbal communication skills in every aspect of education.

Glossary

Feedback — return of information from the receiver that informs the sender of the receiver's reaction

Nonverbal communication — transmission of messages without using words

Social relationship — interaction between two or more people who work together to meet the participants' needs

Therapeutic relationship — interaction between two or more people (such as nurse and patient) who work together to meet at least one participant's needs

Verbal communication — transmission of messages using spoken or written words

Nursing Textbooks

Learning Objectives

After studying this section, the reader should be able to:

● Describe the general format of nursing textbooks and outline strategies for successful reading preparation.

● Discuss the importance of reading for understanding as a way to acquire new knowledge.

● Identify strategies to improve reading comprehension of nursing textbooks.

● Discuss the purpose and format of nursing skillbooks.

● Present strategies for using nursing skillbooks effectively.

VII. Nursing Textbooks

A. Introduction

1. Nursing textbooks differ from general prose such as newspapers, magazines, and novels
2. A student reads nursing textbooks for two reasons
   a. For understanding, to learn new material
   b. For directions, to learn the steps of a clinical skill or procedure
3. A student should prepare for reading assignments to improve comprehension

B. Preparation for reading

1. General information
   a. Nursing textbooks vary in format and level of difficulty according to the aim of the author, the topic presented, and the nature of the intended audience
   b. Despite variations, nursing textbooks share some similarities
   c. Nursing textbooks usually are divided into chapters according to topics
   d. Learning objectives usually are included at the beginning of each chapter
   e. A pre-test to measure prior knowledge may appear at the beginning of each chapter
   f. Key terms and definitions may be listed at the beginning of each chapter
   g. Each chapter usually is written according to a topical outline that is consistent with all other chapters
   h. Boldface topic headings reflect the topical outline of the chapter
   i. Pictures, graphs, and diagrams illustrate and clarify information in the text
   j. Charts and lists summarize information in the text
   k. Nursing care plans may be included to help the student apply theory to nursing practice
   l. A bibliography usually is included at the end of each chapter
   m. A post-test, sample test, or questions to measure learning may follow each chapter
   n. A glossary of terms may be included in each chapter or at the end of the book
   o. Appendices may provide additional information such as case studies, a list of nursing diagnoses, or laboratory values
2. Survival strategies
   a. Scan each textbook to become familiar with its layout
   b. Check for boldface type, highlighted text, italics, charts, and diagrams; these provide clues to what is important in the text
   c. Identify assigned pages
   d. Review learning objectives in the course outline
   e. Read learning objectives at the beginning of the chapter
   f. Identify the focus of the learning objectives and keep it in mind while reading
   g. Skim assigned pages to become familiar with the topic
   h. Note headings and subheadings to become familiar with the chapter's topical outline

      i.   Ask *What is the purpose of this assignment?* and keep formulating the answer while reading

C. Reading textbooks
   1. General information
      a. Textbook reading helps the student acquire new knowledge
      b. New or complex information may be difficult to understand and learn
      c. Textbook reading requires concentration and attentiveness
   2. Survival strategies
      a. Concentrate on reading; less than full attention can impede comprehension of difficult material
      b. Pay attention to definitions, formulas, and examples; they add meaning to the text
      c. Pay attention to diagrams, charts, and illustrations; they help clarify the text
      d. Underline or highlight important information
      e. Make notations in the margin to emphasize important information
      f. Answer review questions at the end of the chapter to evaluate understanding and learning
      g. Identify weak points in understanding; review the appropriate material
      h. Write questions to ask during class for clarification
      i. Summarize the chapter in writing, using paragraph or outline format, to reinforce information and improve retention
      j. Ask *Have I achieved the learning objectives?* to evaluate learning

D. Reading skillbooks
   1. General information
      a. A nursing skillbook is a manual that teaches *how-to* skills
      b. Skills addressed include bedmaking, maintaining sterile technique, and giving injections
      c. A skillbook usually is a companion to a nursing text; for example, the publisher of a nursing fundamentals textbook will publish a related skillbook
      d. A skillbook format will be consistent with its companion textbook format; chapters will be similarly titled and ordered
      e. A skillbook usually includes graphics that illustrate the steps of a particular nursing skill
      f. Each chapter identifies the nursing theory necessary to perform the skill correctly
      g. The procedure for performing a skill is written in step-by-step format
      h. The rationale or theoretical basis for each step explains why the step is necessary
      i. A section on special considerations helps the student understand all implications of the procedure
      j. A checklist for each procedure helps the student evaluate individual performance (see *Sample performance checklist,* page 52)

SAMPLE PERFORMANCE CHECKLIST

SUBCUTANEOUS INJECTION	SATISFACTORY	NEEDS IMPROVEMENT
• Washes hands	☐	☐
• Selects appropriate size and gauge needle and syringe	☐	☐
• Reads medication label when removing container from storage	☐	☐
• Rereads label before withdrawing medication	☐	☐
• Withdraws medication using aseptic technique	☐	☐
• Reads medication label again before discarding the container	☐	☐
• Identifies patient by reading identification band	☐	☐
• Washes hands	☐	☐
• Maintains patient privacy by pulling curtains	☐	☐
• Explains procedure to patient	☐	☐
• Identifies injection site by identifying anatomical landmarks	☐	☐
• Cleans patient's skin with alcohol	☐	☐
• Bunches skin	☐	☐
• Inserts needle at 45 degree angle	☐	☐
• Aspirates to check for blood (unless administering heparin)	☐	☐
• Injects medication	☐	☐
• Removes needle	☐	☐
• Disposes of needle and syringe in puncture-resistant container	☐	☐
• Assists patient to comfortable position	☐	☐
• Washes hands	☐	☐
• Records drug administration on medication record	☐	☐
• Checks patient to evaluate response to medication	☐	☐

2. Survival strategies
   a. Skim the procedure for an overview of the skill
   b. Carefully read each step of the procedure
   c. Pay close attention to pictures and diagrams; they add meaning to the text

d. Try to visualize each step
e. Recite the procedure for each step aloud, paraphrasing the skillbook's language
f. Identify the rationale for each step
g. Practice the skill in the laboratory, following the steps outlined in the skillbook
h. Review and rate actual performance against the performance checklist

Points to Remember

Nursing textbooks vary in scope and level of difficulty, but all have similarities in format.

Preparation for textbook reading includes scanning the chapter for learning objectives, key terms, topic headings, and subheadings.

Charts, diagrams, and illustrations provide information that supports and clarifies the text.

Underline, highlight, or make notes in the margins when reading textbooks to aid recall and review.

Summarizing or outlining the chapter will facilitate learning and improve retention of new information.

Nursing skillbooks supplement textbooks with *how-to* instructions for nursing procedures or skills.

Glossary

Case study — description of a clinical situation, including signs, symptoms, laboratory data, and subjective complaints; used to illustrate application of nursing theory

Nursing care plan — specific plan for nursing care designed to achieve specific outcomes

Nursing diagnosis — definition (using standard nomenclature) of a specific health problem that can be affected by nursing care

Nursing skills — clinical procedures used by nurses, such as measuring vital signs, giving injections, and applying bandages

Pre-test — questions at the beginning of a textbook chapter designed to test existing knowledge about the topic

Nursing Laboratories and Clinical Learning

Learning Objectives

After studying this section, the reader should be able to:

● Describe a nursing laboratory and how it is used in the curriculum.

● Discuss the purpose and identify the location of clinical learning.

● List anxieties common to nursing students in a clinical learning experience.

● Outline strategies to help improve learning in clinical situations.

● Explain the purpose and process of clinical evaluation and how to prepare for it.

VIII. Nursing Laboratories and Clinical Learning

A. Introduction

1. Nursing laboratories are classes in which skills and procedures associated with clinical practice are taught
2. Nursing laboratories provide the opportunity for hands-on practice and demonstration of mastery
3. Clinical learning occurs outside the regular classroom, usually in a health care facility
4. Clinical learning provides an opportunity to apply theory to a practice situation
5. Learning objectives for laboratories and clinical experiences are identified in the course outline; they are directly related to the theory presented in the course

B. Nursing laboratories

1. General information
    a. Nursing laboratories simulate the clinical setting to provide the student with equipment used in nursing practice
    b. Nursing laboratories contain hospital beds and linen, mannequins for practicing patient care, and equipment such as syringes, catheters, and sterile bandages
    c. Skills and procedures may be taught by the laboratory instructor or through audiovisual presentations or computerized instruction programs
    d. The student handles equipment and practices skills in the laboratory under the guidance of an instructor
    e. The laboratory provides a nonthreatening atmosphere for learning and practice
    f. The laboratory provides an opportunity to demonstrate competence before performing a skill in a clinical situation
    g. In addition to teaching skills, the laboratory is the setting for activities such as interviewing and role playing
2. Survival strategies
    a. Complete reading assignments before attending laboratory sessions to become familiar with the skill
    b. Pay attention to demonstrations to understand each step of the procedure
    c. Ask questions as they arise if the instructor is giving the demonstration; at audiovisual presentations, jot down questions to ask later
    d. Practice procedures according to the performance checklist to be sure each step is performed properly
    e. Identify the criteria for measuring competency in the skill to understand how performance will be evaluated (see *Evaluating nursing skills*)
    f. When unable to achieve satisfactory performance, ask the laboratory instructor for assistance and extra time for practice

EVALUATING NURSING SKILLS

The performance of a nursing skill can be measured as competent, satisfactory, or unsatisfactory. Below are behaviors that describe each of these evaluations:

EVALUATION	STUDENT'S BEHAVIORS
Competent	• is prepared and organized • follows the steps outlined in the manual • proceeds independently • demonstrates safe practice and manual dexterity in handling equipment
Satisfactory	• is prepared and organized • needs more practice to develop competence • follows the steps outlined in the manual • demonstrates minimal safe practice or shows awkwardness when handling equipment
Unsatisfactory	• is unprepared and disorganized • lacks self-confidence • needs assistance in order to proceed • fails to follow the steps outlined in the manual • would jeopardize the safety of the patient without supervision • is unsure how to use the equipment

C. Clinical learning
1. General information
   a. Clinical learning provides an opportunity to transfer knowledge from the classroom to a clinical setting
   b. Each student usually spends several weeks during each nursing course in a related clinical setting
   c. Each clinical experience has a specific learning objective that provides focus and direction
   d. Clinical learning provides an opportunity for patient contact, for observing and performing skills, and for practicing problem solving and decision making
   e. The clinical setting provides a learning environment that includes guidance and immediate feedback from the instructor
   f. Clinical learning can take place in various settings, such as hospitals, nursing homes, clinics, ambulatory care centers, and community health centers
   g. The number of hours devoted to clinical learning varies among nursing programs; hours may be daytime or evening

    h. The instructor usually posts patient care assignments the day before the clinical experience

    i. The instructor defines clinical learning objectives and selects patients based on those objectives

    j. The student may need to visit the clinical area the day before the experience to collect patient information

    k. On the day of the clinical experience, the instructor usually holds a preclinical conference to discuss learning objectives and a postclinical conference to review the experience

    l. Written assignments related to the clinical experience may include nursing interviews, nursing care plans, and process recordings

    m. The student may be required to keep a diary or write anecdotal records of clinical learning

    n. The student must evaluate learning and performance and share the evaluation with the instructor

    o. The instructor maintains anecdotal records of each student's clinical performance and provides frequent feedback on strengths and weaknesses

    p. The student may experience stress and anxiety before a clinical experience from a lack of self-confidence, a fear of being incompetent or of harming a patient, or feelings of intimidation from the instructor

  2. Survival strategies

    a. Know the learning objectives for each clinical assignment to make the most of the opportunity

    b. Know school policies on the student's role in the clinical setting, including the limits of a student's duties and responsibilities

    c. Review the clinical evaluation tool to clarify the criteria for evaluating performance; identify behaviors necessary for successful performance

    d. Prepare thoroughly for each clinical assignment: Review patient history, laboratory data, diagnostic tests, medical treatment plan, and nursing care plan

    e. Understand patient care responsibilities; ask questions when unsure

    f. Try to control anxiety, which interferes with learning

    g. Participate in preclinical and postclinical conferences to show interest in learning

    h. Discuss concerns about performance with the instructor for guidance and feedback

D. Clinical evaluation

  1. General information

    a. Informal evaluation, in the form of conversations between student and instructor, takes place during the clinical experience

    b. The instructor observes for behaviors that demonstrate learning objectives; for example, if the objective is to perform a respiratory assessment on a patient, the instructor will look for behaviors such as auscultation of breath sounds and chest examination

c. The instructor writes anecdotal accounts of performance to help make evaluations at the conclusion of the rotation

d. The final clinical evaluation is based on the student's performance during the entire rotation and is rated on an evaluation tool or form.

e. The clinical evaluation tool summarizes learning objectives for each assignment and identifies behaviors that demonstrate successful learning

f. Student and instructor complete separate evaluation tools; when these are compared, both individuals may ask questions and make comments

g. The clinical evaluation should clearly define strengths and weaknesses in clinical performance as well as identify satisfactory or unsatisfactory performance of nursing skills

h. The final evaluation is a formal student-instructor conference during which clinical performance is judged satisfactory (pass) or unsatisfactory (fail) according to specific criteria

i. *Satisfactory* clinical performance is necessary for a student to proceed to the next level nursing course

j. *Unsatisfactory* clinical performance usually results in a failing grade for the entire nursing course

2. Survival strategies

a. Review the clinical evaluation tool throughout the rotation to ensure focus on critical behaviors

b. If the instructor does not give frequent, informal feedback on clinical performance, take the initiative and ask for a discussion

c. Keep an informal diary of each clinical experience; note specific skills or interventions performed to aid in formal self-evaluation

d. Be honest in self-evaluation to help guide future learning experiences

e. Discuss major discrepancies between self-evaluation and the instructor's assessment; use the informal clinical diary for supporting information

Points to Remember

Nursing laboratories simulate clinical settings and provide an opportunity for observing, practicing, and demonstrating competence in clinical skills.

Clinical learning provides an opportunity for patient contact and the application of theory to nursing practice.

A clear understanding of learning objectives and of the limitations of student practice is the best guarantee of successful clinical learning.

Some nervousness is common before a clinical nursing experience, but anxiety should not interfere with the ability to learn.

Glossary

Anecdotal record — informal narrative describing a situation

Clinical learning objective — specific goal or outcome to be achieved during a clinical learning experience

Clinical setting — hospital or other health care agency where the student learns and practices nursing with actual patients

Competence — level of proficiency in essential nursing skills that is acceptable for the safe practice of nursing

Criteria — specific behaviors used as standards on which evaluation is based

Nursing laboratory — class in which nursing skills and procedures are demonstrated by an instructor and practiced by the student; simulates a clinical setting with hospital beds, equipment, and models

Process recording — written verbatim account of verbal interaction between two people for the purpose of analyzing communication; used to help the student learn effective communication skills

Study Skills

Learning Objectives

After studying this section, the reader should be able to:

- Define the four components of studying.

- Explain the importance of a positive attitude toward study.

- Describe the best environment for study.

- Discuss when and how much to study.

- Describe behavior modification as a means to improve memory, concentration, and productivity.

- Identify strategies to improve study skills.

IX. Study Skills

A. Introduction

1. Studying is the process of gathering and learning new information to increase knowledge for use on examinations and in nursing practice
   a. Success in nursing school depends on successful study skills
   b. The development of study skills is enhanced by a positive attitude toward learning
2. Studying involves four activities
   a. Gathering information
   b. Categorizing information
   c. Summarizing information
   d. Storing information for future use
3. Learning is a lifelong process that includes acquiring new ideas and information, rejecting or changing old ideas, and solving problems
   a. Learning can be planned or accidental
   b. Learning can be both fun and hard work
   c. Learning can be hampered by unpleasant memories of previous school experiences, fear of failure, or time constraints

B. Attitude

1. General information
   a. Attitude is an individual's subjective thoughts and feelings about learning
   b. An individual's attitude toward learning is the result of previous experience, which may be positive, negative, or neutral
   c. Every individual should develop a positive attitude toward studying and learning
2. Survival strategies
   a. Plan to take courses in a logical sequence that will build on previously learned information
   b. Stay in control by planning time for study and other commitments
   c. Complete homework and other assignments as soon as possible to avoid falling behind
   d. Anticipate problems and be ready with solutions
   e. Approach each assignment as a challenge
   f. Ask *Why is this important?* to clarify and categorize information
   g. Be competitive by being well-informed and by participating actively in class discussions
   h. Evaluate results of tests and assignments to identify weak points that require extra effort

C. Environment

1. General information
   a. Environment is the place where studying is done
   b. The study environment influences the ability to concentrate on and learn new material

      c. A student can study alone or with a group

      d. The study environment should be clearly labeled as off-limits to those who are not studying

  2. Survival strategies

      a. Establish a separate place to study

      b. Make the study environment comfortable, but not so comfortable that sleep is possible; include a large desk or table, a straight-back chair, and adequate lighting

      c. Equip the study environment with a bookshelf, storage space for paper and supplies, and a large calendar for noting assignments, examinations, and other important dates

      d. Keep the study environment free from distractions such as radio, television, and telephone

      e. Avoid snacking in the study environment, to focus attention and improve concentration

      f. When choosing a study group, select classmates who are capable, serious, and doing well in the course so that group discussion will be productive

      g. Avoid studying with others if a distracting personal relationship is involved

      h. Do not let group study sessions become social occasions

D. Planning study time

  1. General information

      a. Specific hours should be set aside to keep up with course assignments, learn new material, and review old material

      b. Usually, a student should plan 2 hours of study time for each hour in class

      c. Some study each day, rather than 1 or 2 full days of study, improves retention and recall

      d. A student learns more efficiently when study time is planned and the individual is at peak performance level

      e. Family and employment obligations should be considered when planning study time, to use time most efficiently

  2. Survival strategies

      a. Plan to study 2 hours for every class hour to learn new material

      b. Schedule at least 2 to 3 hours of study daily to stay current with reading, assignments, and review

      c. Be realistic when planning study time; fatigue interferes with learning

      d. Plan study for peak performance times to improve concentration and learning

      e. Plan to study when interruption is least likely, to maintain attention and concentration

      f. Try rising early and studying 1 to 2 hours before the household awakes or scheduled commitments begin, to avoid distractions and interruptions

g. Start each study session with the most difficult subject or task to be as alert as possible

h. If studying when tired, choose subjects that require the least concentration

i. For maximum efficiency, limit an uninterrupted study session to 2 hours

j. Schedule short breaks between subjects to avoid fatigue

k. Use time before and after class to review notes

E. Behavior modification
1. General information
    a. Behavior modification is a conscious attempt to change behavior for specific results
    b. Behavior modification can be used to improve study skills and learning
    c. Behavior modification techniques to improve study skills include setting deadlines, giving oneself rewards, performing memory exercises, analyzing tasks, participating in study groups, and seeking help
    d. A student who sets and meets deadlines becomes goal-directed and more efficient
    e. Rewards for completing a task or assignment increase motivation
    f. Memory exercises improve information retention and recall
    g. Task analysis defines the extent of an assignment and the time required to complete it
    h. Participation in study groups where concepts and theories are verbalized improves information retention and recall
2. Survival strategies
    a. Set deadlines for completing tasks; determine to meet deadlines consistently
    b. If concentrating is difficult, break tasks into smaller units and set short-term goals; for example, reading six pages in 20 minutes
    c. Record each day's study time; try to increase it gradually
    d. When concentrating fails, take a 5 to 10 minute break
    e. Participate regularly in enjoyable activities so that study does not become a burden
    f. Reward successful completion of tasks; plan long-term rewards for completing long or difficult assignments (schedule an evening with a friend, for example)
    g. Do not feel guilty about deviating from the study schedule; make adjustments as needed and try again
    h. Share study plans with spouse, children, friends, and significant others to gain understanding and support
    i. Set aside specific time for family and friends
    j. Be sensitive to others' needs, but firm in the commitment to study
    k. Learn to reject requests and invitations that interfere with study

l. Be flexible; adjust study schedule when necessary, but not to the point of falling behind in course work

m. Be enthusiastic; view learning as a challenge

n. Personalize information: Ask *How will I use this?* to improve recall

o. Use acronyms and mnemonics to help memorize data; for example, ABC is the acronym for airway, breathing, and circulation

p. Use imagination to improve memory: Illustrate notes with sketches; read aloud to use listening skills; create mental images of text; exaggerate information to make it more memorable

q. Analyze assignments to plan time; for example, determine if library work, research, a laboratory, or clinical experience is involved

r. Identify conflicting commitments and assignments; plan time accordingly

s. Seek help from instructors and tutors to avoid feeling overwhelmed

Points to Remember

Studying is the process of gathering new information and committing it to memory for recall and use.

Curiosity and a competitive attitude will enhance learning.

Studying is most efficient and effective in a quiet place without distractions or interruptions.

Two to three hours of study should be scheduled each school day to improve information retention and recall.

Behavior can be modified to improve motivation for study, concentration, memorization, and recall.

Glossary

Acronym — a word formed from the first letters of a compound term or phrase; for example, NANDA is the acronym for North American Nursing Diagnosis Association

Behavior modification — specific techniques used to change behavior

Mnemonic — a device or code used to help remember a complicated concept or list of information; for example, On Old Olympus's Towering Tops, A Finn And German Viewed Some Hops is a mnemonic device for remembering the order of the Cranial nerves (O-olfactory; O-optic; O-oculomotor; T-trochlear; T-trigeminal; A-abdurens; F-facial; A-acoustic; G-glossopharyngeal; V-vagus; S-spinal accessory; H-hypoglossal)

Study group — several students who meet regularly to review and discuss course content

Task analysis — examination of a task to identify its component parts and the skills that will be needed to complete it

Taking Examinations

Learning Objectives
After studying this section, the reader should be able to:

- Describe the three domains of learning.

- List the learning domains measured by objective, essay, and oral examinations.

- Discuss strategies to use when preparing for an examination.

- Identify the kinds of questions that may be asked on an examination.

- Present strategies for answering each kind of examination question.

- Discuss strategies to use when taking an examination.

X. Taking Examinations

A. Introduction

1. Examinations or tests are evaluation methods used to measure learning
   a. Nursing students are required to take examinations in nonnursing courses, such as anatomy, chemistry, and sociology, as well as in nursing courses
   b. Nursing theory and nursing skills examinations are different from non-nursing examinations (see Section XI for more information)
2. Learning occurs in three domains: cognitive, affective, and psychomotor
   a. The *cognitive* domain involves comprehension, application, analysis, synthesis, and evaluation
   b. Cognitive learning is most easily measured by written or oral examinations
   c. The *affective* domain involves attitudes and values related to the learning content
   d. Affective learning is measured by behavior; it is not easily measured by examinations
   e. The *psychomotor* domain involves performing a skill or procedure
   f. Psychomotor learning is best measured by demonstration or performance of the skill or procedure
3. Examinations test learning in each domain; they may be written or oral
4. Written examinations can be objective tests or essay tests
5. *Objective* examinations measure learning in the cognitive and psychomotor domains
   a. Objective examinations test knowledge, comprehension, application, synthesis, and evaluation
   b. Objective examinations usually are used in large classes; they are easy to administer and can be corrected by a teaching assistant or a computer
   c. Objective examinations can include true-false and multiple choice questions, identification, matching tests, and sentence completion
6. *Essay* examinations measure learning in the cognitive and affective domains
   a. Essay examinations can measure attitudes and values as well as knowledge
   b. Essay examinations usually are used in smaller classes, such as seminars; they take more time to correct than objective examinations
   c. Essay examinations may be graded by the course instructor or a teaching assistant
7. *Oral* examinations measure learning in the cognitive and affective domains
   a. Oral examinations can measure attitudes and values as well as knowledge
   b. Oral examinations usually are used in small classes or seminars; they typically involve a class presentation
   c. Oral examinations usually are graded by the course instructor

B. Preparing for examinations
1. General information
   a. The most reliable preparation for any examination is to keep up with course work and review notes frequently
   b. Adequate preparation helps ease test-taking anxiety
   c. Test questions are designed to measure learning as outlined in course or unit objectives
2. Survival strategies
   a. Keep up with reading assignments and review class notes daily to avoid falling behind in course work and to reinforce information
   b. Memorize formulas, equivalents, and similar material; review frequently
   c. Practice math problems regularly
   d. Ask the instructor what the examination will cover, and review course and unit objectives to focus study
   e. Ask the instructor which kinds of questions will be asked
   f. Prepare a study schedule that allows time to review without interfering with other courses
   g. Try to anticipate examination questions based on material that was emphasized in class assignments and discussions
   h. Discuss possible questions with classmates
   i. Begin by studying the most difficult material; progress to easier material
   j. Spend minimal time on familiar material
   k. Avoid cramming; it increases anxiety and interferes with learning
   l. The night before an examination, review notes for 1 to 2 hours to refresh memory and facilitate recall
   m. Gather supplies—such as #2 pencils, pens, eraser, calculator, and scratch paper—in advance to avoid rushing before the examination
   n. Relax and get sufficient sleep the night before the examination
   o. Avoid stimulants such as caffeine and other drugs that can interfere with alertness and clear thinking
   p. On the day of the examination, allow extra time for preparation and travel to avoid rushing or being late
   q. Eat a meal that will prevent distraction from hunger during the examination
   r. Arrive at the examination room early enough to sit away from distractions; avoid sitting near friends if they will distract
C. Taking examinations
1. General information
   a. Examinations usually are given within specific time limits
   b. The time allotted depends on whether the examination is objective, essay, or oral
   c. Examinations given at the end of courses (final examinations) usually are allotted more time than others because they are more comprehensive

      d. Final examinations usually are scheduled during a separate examination week

      e. The frequency of examinations is determined by the instructor: Some courses may have only a midterm and a final examination; others may have examinations periodically throughout the term

2. Survival strategies: General

      a. Know how much time is allotted for the examination to plan proper pacing

      b. Ask if unanswered questions are graded as incorrect

      c. Read directions carefully; ask the instructor or monitor for clarifications before beginning

      d. Review the entire examination before starting to allocate time for each section

      e. Answer the easiest questions first to gain confidence and avoid feeling frustrated and anxious; go back to more difficult questions

      f. When unsure of an answer in an examination in which unanswered questions are graded as incorrect, make a guess

      g. Watch for instructor give-aways; for example, the answer to one question is sometimes found in another question

      h. Concentrate on one question at a time

      i. Work as quickly as possible

      j. Try not to skip questions when using a separate answer sheet; an answer marked after the wrong number may result

      k. Concentrate on the examination; wandering attention wastes time

      l. After answering every question, reread the examination to double-check responses

      m. Do not hesitate to change an answer upon reconsideration

      n. After taking an examination, forget about it until it is graded; worrying causes anxiety and stress

      o. Review the graded examination; note errors and weaknesses for future study and motivation

      p. Note the kinds of questions asked and the way in which essay questions were graded to help plan for future examinations

3. Survival strategies: Objective, essay, and oral examinations

      a. Read multiple-choice and true-false questions carefully to be sure of what is being asked

      b. Try to answer multiple-choice questions mentally before looking at the choices; choose that answer if it is among the options

      c. If that answer is not among the options, reread each option carefully to begin eliminating incorrect ones

      d. If an option is incorrect, cross it out and go on to the next one

      e. For each option, look for qualifying words such as *always, all, never, none*; such absolutes commonly make statements incorrect

      f. Avoid reading information into a question that could alter its meaning

g. Do not leave a question unanswered; narrow the choices, then make the best possible guess

h. With true-false questions, watch for words such as *all, always, never, only* that usually make the statement false

i. Read *essay questions* carefully; look for key words that will help focus the answer correctly

j. When the question asks for *comparison*, stress *resemblances* in the answer

k. When the question asks for *contrast*, stress *differences* in the answer

l. When the question asks for *criticism*, express *judgment* in the answer

m. When the question asks for *definition*, provide *clear descriptions and meaning* in the answer

n. When the question asks for *discussion*, examine issues thoroughly and present *pros and cons* in the answer

o. When the question asks for *evaluation*, give an *appraisal* in the answer

p. When the question asks for *explanation, clarify* and *interpret* the issue in the answer

q. Before writing the essay, organize the answer on scratch paper; list major points and supporting data

r. Begin the essay with a direct answer to provide focus and establish a position

s. Give an overview of the main points in the next paragraph, with statements supporting each point to demonstrate knowledge and logical thinking

t. Avoid long, rambling sentences

u. Avoid writing too much

v. When unsure of the answer, begin with as many fragments of information as possible to help jog memory

w. Write legibly or print

x. Practice *oral presentations* in front of a mirror or a friend to gain confidence

y. At an oral examination, think before speaking; speak clearly and avoid rambling

Points to Remember

Examinations may be objective, essay, or oral; they measure learning in the cognitive, affective, and psychomotor domains.

The surest way to prepare for examinations is to keep up with course assignments and study regularly.

Extra time for study and review should be part of preparation for examinations.

On a multiple-choice examination, read questions carefully and examine the options given to make the best choice.

Organize answers to essay questions before beginning to write. Answer questions directly and concisely, using supporting data as necessary.

Glossary

Comprehension — level of cognitive learning involving the understanding of information and the ability to draw conclusions

Multiple-choice question — a statement followed by several options, one of which is the correct answer; used on an objective examination

Synthesis — level of cognitive learning built on knowledge, comprehension, application, and analysis; involves assembling elements of information to create a new idea

Test anxiety — fear of taking examinations; usually includes fear of the unknown and lack of knowledge, preparation, and self-confidence

Nursing Examinations

Learning Objectives

After studying this section, the reader should be able to:

- Explain the purpose of nursing theory examinations.

- Describe the kinds of questions found on nursing theory examinations.

- Discuss strategies to use when taking nursing theory examinations.

- Explain the purpose of nursing skills examinations.

- Describe the kinds of questions found on nursing skills examinations.

- Discuss strategies to use when taking nursing skills examinations.

XI. Nursing Examinations

A. Introduction

1. Nursing examinations test knowledge, judgment, and skills and determine competency in nursing practice
2. Most nursing examinations are objective, using multiple-choice questions
3. Nursing examinations provide the student with practice for taking the National Council Licensure Examination for Registered Nurses (NCLEX-RN) (see Appendix C, Sample NCLEX-RN Questions)
4. Nursing examinations test practical knowledge and skills as well as theoretical knowledge

B. Nursing theory examinations

1. General information
   a. Nursing theory examinations measure learning in the cognitive, affective, and psychomotor domains
   b. Objective examinations measure learning and knowledge and are used to determine competency in a course; they are the most frequently used examinations in nursing
   c. Objective questions that measure learning in the *cognitive* domain usually demand recall of information (see *Sample examination questions, example #1*)
   d. Objective questions that measure learning in the *affective* domain require the ability to apply knowledge to a clinical situation by analyzing information and drawing conclusions (see example #2)
   e. Objective questions that measure learning in the *cognitive* and *affective* domains require the ability to make judgments (see example #3)
   f. Objective questions can measure learning in the *psychomotor* domain and require the ability to demonstrate knowledge of the procedure, sequence of steps, and rationale for each step (see example #4)
   g. Essay questions also can measure nursing knowledge, but are not widely used because of the difficulty of objectively grading written answers for large numbers of students
2. Survival strategies
   a. Keep up with course reading to avoid feeling overwhelmed when preparing for a nursing examination
   b. Read each question carefully to understand what is being asked
   c. Consider each option separately; avoid choosing one only because it looks familiar
   d. When more than one option seems correct, reexamine each one carefully; then select the *one best* answer among the choices
   e. Pay careful attention to *all* information in the case study; the question is designed to test the ability to use all available data

SAMPLE EXAMINATION QUESTIONS

Below are samples of questions commonly found on nursing examinations. Each question tests a different area of knowledge and learning.

1. Testing knowledge

Amphotericin B is usually administered
   A. Orally
   B. Topically
   C. Intramuscularly
   D. Intravenously

This question measures information recall. It does not require high-level thinking or analysis, but it does require the ability to recognize the correct answer based on information from lectures or reading.

2. Testing application of knowledge to a clinical situation

Mrs. Brown, 86 years old, is admitted to the hospital with a medical diagnosis of pneumonia. She complains of weakness and dyspnea, weighs 96 lbs (43.5 kg), and is febrile.

Mrs. Brown maintains a high Fowler's position to ease her breathing. Which body pressure areas are at risk for altered skin integrity?
   A. Malleolus, greater trochanter, ear
   B. Heels, sacrum, elbows
   C. Heels, ischial tuberosity, sacrum
   D. Toes, patellae, acromial process

This question requires information recall about Fowler's position, body pressure areas, and the process of skin breakdown. It also requires information about the patient's ability to move, which is significant in this situation. The student will use recall knowledge and information in the situation to help arrive at the correct answer.

3. Testing the ability to make judgments

Mrs. Smith, a 75-year-old widow, is diagnosed with advanced stomach cancer. She is scheduled for surgery, which she knows is not curative, but which may prolong her life. Before surgery, Mrs. Smith states that she has changed her mind: She does not want to have surgery. She explains that she has had a long and happy life and is not afraid of death. She asks her nurse to help her decide what to do. The nurse believes that all available medical treatment should be used to prolong Mrs. Smith's life. This nurse should:
   A. Ask for a change in assignment
   B. Tell Mrs. Smith that she should have the surgery
   C. Ask Mrs. Smith's family to convince her to have surgery
   D. Acknowledge the patient's right to decide what is best for her, and her right to change her mind. Assure her that care will be available in any event

This question measures learning in communication skills, nurse-patient relationships, advocacy, patient teaching, stress adaptation, and decision making. In addition to measuring information recall, it measures the ability to synthesize information and to make judgments.

continued

SAMPLE EXAMINATION QUESTIONS continued

4. Testing knowledge of how to perform a skill

Identify the proper sequence for preparing injectable medication from a multidose vial.
1. Pull back the plunger to obtain the correct amount of medication
2. Clean the surface of the vial with an alcohol sponge
3. Inject air into the vial
4. Invert the vial
5. Tap the syringe to dislodge any air bubbles
6. Remove the needle from the vial
   A. 1, 2, 3, 5, 6, 4
   B. 2, 3, 4, 1, 5, 6
   C. 2, 4, 5, 1, 3, 6
   D. 2, 1, 3, 5, 4, 6

This question requires recall of the proper sequence for performing this skill. It does *not* test physical performance of the skill, which usually is done by requiring return demonstration of the skill in a nursing practice examination.

 f. Avoid reading any information into the case study; base answers on only the information given

 g. Review graded examinations for weaknesses to improve before the next examination

 h. Consider each nursing examination as practice for the NCLEX-RN (see Section XIV for additional strategies)

C. Nursing skills examinations
 1. General information
  a. Nursing, or *fundamental*, skills are techniques and procedures associated with the clinical practice of nursing
  b. Step-by-step procedures for nursing skills are described in nursing skill books, demonstrated in films and videotapes, and practiced in nursing laboratories
  c. Each nursing skill involves critical elements or behaviors
  d. Nursing skills are tested to assure basic competence and safety in clinical practice
  e. Injections, sterile technique, intravenous therapy and indwelling urinary catheter insertion are some of the fundamental skills necessary for nursing practice
  f. Nursing skill examinations usually take place in the nursing laboratory, but also may be held in the clinical area with patients
 2. Survival strategies
  a. Know which skills will be tested, and review clinical objectives to focus study and practice time

b. Read procedures carefully and ask questions of the instructor to clarify understanding

c. Review the performance checklist to identify critical elements required to perform the skill

d. Practice the skill using the performance checklist to ensure all critical elements are included

e. Reread the procedure outlined in the nursing skillbook to increase familiarity with the procedure

f. Concentrate on why the procedure is done and what it requires rather than using rote memory

g. Ask a classmate to critique performance before clinical testing to gain self-confidence and reduce anxiety

h. Remain calm; avoid listening to rumors and classmates' opinions to maximize concentration and decrease anxiety

Points to Remember

Nursing examinations measure knowledge necessary for the competent and safe practice of nursing.

Nursing theory examinations usually are objective, multiple-choice tests whose format is the same as that for the NCLEX-RN.

Preparation for nursing theory examinations includes keeping up with course work through consistent study and preparation of assignments and reviewing class notes regularly.

Nursing skills examinations test basic competency in the techniques and procedures of nursing practice.

Preparation for nursing skills examinations includes studying procedures, viewing media, and practicing skills.

Glossary

Case study — example of a clinical situation, including signs, symptoms, feelings, and behaviors, used to measure the ability to apply theoretical knowledge in a clinical setting

Judgment — ability to make appropriate decisions and act on those decisions

Nursing skills examination — test given to measure performance of procedures according to specific criteria

Nursing theory examination — test given to evaluate knowledge and competency in meeting nursing course objectives

Time Management

Learning Objectives

After studying this section, the reader should be able to:

- Define time management.

- Explain the importance of time management for a student.

- Identify the elements necessary for time management.

- Discuss strategies for managing time effectively.

XII. Time Management

A. Introduction

1. Time management is the efficient use of time to meet all obligations and achieve specific objectives
2. The way a student uses time influences the ability to prepare for classes, complete assignments, and review for examinations
3. Time management requires identifying family, employment, school, social, and other obligations
4. Time management involves setting priorities, estimating time needed for each task, and developing a schedule (see *Sample time management schedule*)

B. Setting priorities

1. General information
   a. Establishing priorities is the first step toward effective time management
   b. Assigning priorities to commitments is influenced by personal goals
   c. Setting priorities involves identifying obligations and ranking them according to importance
2. Survival strategies
   a. List must-do activities such as work, meal preparation, children's lessons, appointments, and classes to identify regular obligations
   b. List secondary activities such as volunteer work, social events, entertaining, and shopping to identify additional time demands
   c. Recruit others for tasks such as household chores
   d. Decide which activities are essential and which can be postponed or eliminated
   e. List all personal obligations; remember them when preparing weekly schedule

C. Estimating time

1. General information
   a. Estimating time involves planning for priorities such as study, work, and home commitments
   b. Estimating time requires being realistic; consider abilities and past experience when alloting time for school and study
   c. The general rule for calculating study time is two hours of study for each hour of class
   d. Actual time needed for study varies according to difficulty of the subject, prior knowledge of the subject, and personal interest in it
2. Survival strategies
   a. Analyze assignments to plan sufficient time for each task
   b. Plan time for textbook reading to keep up with course material
   c. Plan time for outside readings and research
   d. Plan time for typing and photocopying
   e. Plan time to prepare written assignments, care plans, and self-evaluation
   f. Plan time to prepare group presentations, projects, and oral reports

SAMPLE TIME MANAGEMENT SCHEDULE

	MONDAY	TUESDAY	WEDNESDAY	THURSDAY	FRIDAY	SATURDAY	SUNDAY
6:00-7:00 A.M.	Family breakfast	Family breakfast	Family breakfast	Family breakfast	Family breakfast	Family breakfast	Family breakfast
7:00-8:00 A.M.	Commute	Commute	Commute	Commute	Commute	Household chores and errands	Family
8:00-9:00 A.M.	Nursing	Nursing Lab	Nursing	Study	Clinical		
9:00-10:00 A.M.	↓	English Comp	↓	English Comp			
10:00-11:00 A.M.	Math for Pharma-cology	↓	Math for Pharma-cology	↓			
11:00 A.M.-12:00 P.M.	↓	↓	↓	↓			
12:00-1:00 P.M.	Lunch	Lunch	Lunch	Lunch			
1:00-2:00 P.M.	Study	Study	Study	Commute			↓
2:00-3:00 P.M.	Commute	Commute	Commute	Clinical assignment	↓	↓	Study
3:00-4:00 P.M.	Exercise class	Exercise class	Exercise class	Exercise class	Exercise class	Study	↓
4:00-5:00 P.M.	Family and dinner	Family and dinner	Family and dinner	Family and dinner	Family and dinner	Family and dinner	↓
5:00-6:00 P.M.	↓	↓	↓	↓	↓	↓	Dinner and family time
6:00-7:00 P.M.	Organize household	Organize household	Organize household	Organize household	Time off	Time off	↓
7:00-8:00 P.M.	Study	Study	Study	Prepare for clinical	↓	↓	↓
8:00-9:00 P.M.	↓	↓	↓	↓	↓	↓	Study
9:00-10:00 P.M.	Time with spouse	Time with spouse	Time with spouse	Time with spouse	Time with spouse	Time with spouse	Time with spouse
10:00 P.M.-6:00 A.M.	Sleep	Sleep	Sleep	Sleep	Sleep	Sleep	Sleep

g. Plan time for data collection at the clinical site before a clinical experience

h. Plan time for clinical learning preparation such as reviewing patient diagnosis, pathophysiology, nursing diagnosis, and drugs; and developing a nursing care plan

i. Plan time for travel to school and clinical sites

D. Scheduling
1. General information
   a. A schedule is a plan of action for a specific time period
   b. A schedule reflects priorities, with the most important activities accorded the most time
   c. A schedule shows time estimated for each task
   d. A schedule should include family, work, and social commitments as well as school assignments, tests, and study periods
   e. A schedule should be realistic, allowing for unexpected variables
2. Survival strategies
   a. Use a large calendar to plan the entire semester
   b. Record firmly committed periods such as class, laboratory, and clinic times
   c. Record examination dates and due dates for assignments
   d. Record employment and social obligations
   e. Identify free time periods
   f. Schedule school and home study time during free periods; alert family members to at-home study times to avoid interruptions
   g. Use time between classes for review and preparation
   h. Be realistic; failure to meet an overambitious schedule can result in guilt and frustration
   i. Be flexible; a week or two into the semester, adjust the schedule as necessary
   j. Schedule extra time for difficult subjects; do not steal time from one subject to work on another
   k. When overwhelmed, falling behind, or physically exhausted, review the schedule and seek advice from an academic counselor
   l. Schedule study for peak performance times
   m. Schedule frequent short study periods rather than occasional long sessions for easier incorporation into a daily routine
   n. Schedule study time each day (see *Sample weekly study schedule*)
   o. Schedule time for rest and relaxation to avoid overwork and stress

SAMPLE WEEKLY STUDY SCHEDULE

Below is a sample of a weekly study schedule for a student with a course load of 17 credit hours. This schedule shows 30 hours of planned study. The student should record actual study hours.

DAY	CLASS TIME	PLANNED STUDY HOURS	ACTUAL STUDY HOURS
Monday	8:00 - 10:00 A.M. 12:00 - 1:00 P.M.	10:00 - 11:30 A.M. 3:00 - 5:00 P.M. 7:00 - 9:00 P.M.	
Tuesday	9:00 - 12:00 NOON 12:30 - 2:30 P.M.	8:00 - 9:00 A.M. 7:00 - 10:00 P.M.	
Wednesday	8:00 - 10:00 A.M. 12:00 - 1:00 P.M.	10:00 - 11:30 A.M. 3:00 - 5:00 P.M. 7:00 - 9:00 P.M.	
Thursday	9:00 - 12:00 NOON	8:00 - 9:00 A.M. 7:00 - 10:00 P.M.	
Friday	8:00 - 10:00 A.M. 12:00 - 1:00 P.M.	10:00 - 11:30 A.M. 3:00 - 5:00 P.M. 7:00 - 9:00 P.M.	
Saturday		3:00 - 5:00 P.M.	
Sunday		3:00 - 5:00 P.M. 7:30 - 9:00 P.M.	

Points to Remember

Time management is the efficient use of time to meet obligations and achieve goals.

To manage time effectively, a student must identify obligations and list them according to priority.

Preparing a daily schedule of class times, study times, and other obligations helps manage time effectively.

Time management schedules should be realistic, allow for variables, and be adjusted periodically.

Glossary

Time management — efficient use of time to meet obligations and achieve goals

Priority — degree of importance assigned to an obligation

Schedule — written plan for a specified period of time

Stress Management

Learning Objectives

After studying this section, the reader should be able to:

- Define stress.

- Discuss the major sources of stress for nursing students and the effect of stress on learning.

- Identify the physical, emotional, and social symptoms of stress.

- Describe techniques for stress reduction.

XIII. Stress Management

A. Introduction

1. Stress is a state of physical or mental tension that results from physical, chemical, or emotional factors
2. The body responds to positive and negative stimuli, called stressors
   a. Examples of positive stressors are happy occasions such as a wedding or job promotion
   b. Examples of negative stressors are unhappy occasions such as the loss of a job or death of a loved one
   c. Positive and negative stressors are a normal part of life and play an important role in emotional growth and development
3. Depending on its degree, stress can have a positive or negative effect on learning.
   a. In some instances, when the level is low, stress can be a motivator for learning
   b. However, increasing levels of stress can interfere with learning
4. Sources of stress for nursing students include physical and emotional demands of school and professional concerns
5. Physical sources of stress include:
   a. Studying
   b. Standing, lifting clients, and moving equipment
   c. Attending class and studying when ill to avoid falling behind
6. Emotional sources of stress include:
   a. Fear of the unknown or of failure
   b. Anxiety about assignments, tests, or clinical practice
   c. Insecurity about the ability to succeed
   d. Guilt over mistakes, poor evaluations, or low grades
   e. Competitiveness
   f. Separation from family or friends
7. Professional sources of stress include:
   a. Anxiety about performance in the professional role
   b. Fear of forgetting important information or skills
   c. Fear of inflicting pain on, or otherwise harming, a patient
   d. Feelings of intimidation about more experienced classmates
   e. Anxiety about meeting the expectations of an instructor
   f. Worry about coping with terminally ill patients
8. A student may respond to stressors physically, emotionally, or through social behavior
9. Physical responses to stressors include:
   a. Increased or decreased appetite
   b. Increased junk food consumption
   c. Excessive alcohol consumption
   d. Excessive smoking

e. Drug abuse
f. Stomachache, diarrhea, constipation
g. Dry mouth, sweaty palms
h. Trembling, tics, twitches, muscle spasms
i. Teeth grinding, jaw clenching
j. Nail biting
k. Chronic fatigue, insomnia, nightmares
l. Headache
m. Impaired sexual function

10. Emotional responses to stressors include:
   a. Crying
   b. Complaining
   c. Anger, hostility
   d. Irritability
   e. Mistrust
   f. Mood swings
   g. Constant worrying about school or job

11. Social responses to stressors include:
   a. Quarreling
   b. Blaming others
   c. Criticizing others
   d. Being unable to relax with others
   e. Dominating conversations by talking exclusively about school or other sources of stress
   f. Withdrawing from family and friends

B. Stress management
1. General information
   a. Identifying stressors and assessing stress level is the first step in stress management
   b. Maintaining a healthy body helps manage stress
   c. Practicing relaxation techniques helps control harmful effects of stress
   d. Developing a positive attitude helps reduce the frustration and disappointments associated with stress
   e. Maintaining a social support system helps control stress
   f. Maintaining a spiritual dimension can counterbalance stress
2. Survival strategies
   a. Exercise regularly to improve strength and tolerance for the physical demands of nursing
   b. Get adequate sleep to maintain stamina and health
   c. Eat a balanced diet to meet the body's need for nutrients
   d. Limit junk food and alcohol to avoid the effects of stimulants and depressants

e. Quit smoking to avoid impairing respiratory and cardiac function
f. Use medication only as prescribed to maintain clear thinking
g. Practice muscle relaxation and breathing exercises to reduce tension
h. Practice imaging, meditation, or yoga for relaxation and improved mental and physical performance
i. Develop a positive attitude to improve emotional health
j. Use energy for problem solving, not self-pity
k. View problems from a long-term perspective; ask *How important will this be 5 years from now?* to develop a realistic outlook
l. Don't anticipate problems; handle them as they arise
m. Develop a sense of humor
n. Express emotions to release tension
o. Work off anger with physical exercise
p. Maintain social support systems to help during difficult times
q. Share both good and bad news with family and friends to ensure continuing support
r. Improve or end troubled relationships
s. Engage in diversions such as hobbies and entertainment
t. Maintain a spiritual dimension; pray, meditate, or attend religious services
u. Do something thoughtful for another person to give meaning to values and beliefs.
v. Seek counseling when feeling overwhelmed by stress

Points to Remember

The physical and emotional demands of nursing school, as well as professional concerns, are sources of stress for nursing students.

The body's response to everyday stresses can be expressed physicallly, emotionally, or socially.

Maintaining a healthy body, practicing relaxation techniques, and developing a positive attitude are ways to help cope with negative stress.

Glossary

Breathing exercise — technique based on conscious and controlled inhaling and exhaling; with practice, a slow, regular breathing pattern is achieved and tension is reduced, thereby limiting the body's response to stress

Imaging — technique used to call to mind a specific pleasant scene or event on which the individual concentrates until distractions are excluded

Meditation — mental exercise that uses concentrating on a single thought, idea, or focus for a short time to eliminate distractions from consciousness, resulting in sharpened concentration

Muscle relaxation exercise — conscious technique to ease tension in various body parts until the entire body is relaxed; with practice, can be used to control stress at will

Stress — a state of physical or mental tension that results from physical, mental, or emotional factors

Yoga — meditation technique practiced to attain higher consciousness, allowing one to move beyond a stressful situation to a tranquil state

After Graduation

Learning Objectives

After studying this section, the reader should be able to:

● Define licensure.

● Explain the significance of the nurse practice act as it relates to licensure.

● List the key components of licensing laws.

● Discuss the National Council Licensure Examination for Registered Nurses (NCLEX-RN).

● Identify the major categories of the NCLEX-RN.

● Describe strategies to prepare for and take the NCLEX-RN.

XIV. After Graduation

A. Introduction

1. The approach of graduation from a nursing program generates excitement
   a. The student is fulfilling long-term goals
   b. The student anticipates starting a new career
   c. The student is about to use knowledge gained through classroom and clinical learning
2. Graduation is not the final step
3. To practice nursing, the student must meet two requirements
   a. Licensure
   b. Successful completion of the National Council Licensure Examination for Registered Nurses (NCLEX-RN) (see Appendix C, Sample NCLEX-RN Questions)

B. Licensure

1. General information
   a. Licensure is the legal mechanism that regulates the practice of nursing
   b. A nursing license entitles an individual to practice as a professionally qualified nurse
   c. Licensure is designed to safeguard the public and hold nurses accountable for their practice
   d. Licensure is required for the practice of nursing in the United States and Canada
   e. Licensure is regulated by agencies called boards of nursing
   f. In the United States, each state has a board of nursing; in Canada, each province has one
   g. Each board of nursing establishes a nurse practice act
   h. Nurse practice acts are designed to protect the public by broadly defining the legal scope of nursing practice
   i. Licensing laws are contained within nurse practice acts
   j. Licensing laws establish the requirements for obtaining and maintaining a nursing license
2. Key components of licensing laws
   a. Requirements for licensing, such as completion of basic professional nursing education program and NCLEX-RN, good moral character, residency
   b. License application procedures and reciprocal licensing arrangements
   c. Application fees
   d. Authorization for applicants who receive licenses to use the title Registered Nurse (RN)
   e. Grounds for license denial, revocation, or suspension
   f. License renewal procedures
3. Survival strategies
   a. Obtain a copy of the state's or province's nurse practice act, and review it carefully

    b. Know the requirements for licensure

    c. Seek assistance from nursing program faculty about application procedures

    d. Contact the state board of nursing with questions about requirements well before graduation to avoid delay in licensure

C. NCLEX-RN

  1. General information

    a. Graduation from nursing school is an important step toward realizing one's career goal of becoming an RN

    b. To practice as an RN, the student must first pass the NCLEX-RN

    c. NCLEX-RN is the licensing examination used in all fifty states to test for minimum competency in nursing practice

    d. The National Council of State Boards of Nursing has identified behaviors that are critical for the safe and effective practice of nursing

    e. A candidate wishing to take the examination must apply to the state in which he or she intends to practice

    f. NCLEX-RN is offered twice yearly, in July and February; it is administered over a two-day period

    g. In the past, the test was grouped according to specialties, such as medical, surgical, pediatric, maternal, and psychiatric nursing; today, it consists of four 90-minute integrated segments

    h. NCLEX-RN contains approximately 375 multiple choice questions; a new examination is developed for each test date

    i. The content of the examination is based on nursing practice

    j. Questions follow a test plan or blueprint that organizes content into two broad categories: the nursing process and patient (client) needs

    k. Each question matches one phase of the nursing process and one type of patient need (See *Nursing process* and *Patient needs,* page 95)

    l. Questions test knowledge, skills, and traits necessary for safe practice

    m. Questions are based on health care situations in which decision making is shared by or centered on the nurse or the patient

    n. Candidates receive test results approximately 6 to 8 weeks after taking the test

    o. A passing score is 1,600 out of a possible 3,200; test results are reported as "pass" or "fail"

    p. Unsuccessful candidates receive a diagnostic profile indicating areas failed and how far performance fell short of the passing mark

  2. Survival strategies

    a. Prepare for NCLEX-RN from the first day of nursing school; pay careful attention to all nursing examinations, which are similar in design to NCLEX-RN

    b. Develop test-taking skills by learning from experience

NURSING PROCESS

The chart below lists the five phases of the nursing process with specific behaviors associated with each phase, as measured by the National Council Licensure Examination for Registered Nurses.

NURSING PROCESS PHASE	BEHAVIORS
Assessing—establishing a data base and gathering objective and subjective information	• Collect information from verbal and nonverbal interactions with patient, family and friends, health team members, records, and other pertinent sources • Examine standard data sources for information • Recognize symptoms and findings • Determine the patient's ability to assume personal care of daily health needs • Assess the patient's environment • Identify your reactions to the patient • Confirm observations or perceptions by obtaining additional information • As indicated, question orders and decisions by other staff members • Personally check the patient's condition, instead of relying solely on equipment • Communicate information gained in patient assessment
Analyzing—identifying actual or potential health care needs or problems	• Interpret, validate, and organize data • Collect additional data as indicated • Identify and communicate the patient's nursing diagnoses • Determine congruency between the patient's needs and the health care team's ability to meet those needs
Planning—setting goals to meet the patient's needs and designing strategies to achieve these goals	• In setting goals, involve patient, family and friends, and other health care team members • Establish priorities among goals • Anticipate needs on the basis of established priorities *Develop and modify patient care plan* • Involve the patient, family and friends, or other health care team members in designing care strategies • Include all the information needed to manage the patient's condition • Plan for the patient's comfort and maintenance of optimal functioning • Select appropriate nursing measures to deliver effective patient care *Collaborate with other health care personnel to delivery appropriate care* • Identify health agencies and social resources in the community to assist the patient and patient's family • Coordinate care for the patient's benefit • Delegate responsibilities to other health care providers • Formulate expected outcomes of nursing interventions

continued

NURSING PROCESS continued

NURSING PROCESS PHASE	BEHAVIORS
Implementing— initiating and completing actions necessary to accomplish defined goals	• Organize and manage the patient's care • Perform or assist in performing activities of daily living • Institute measures to provide comfort for the patient • Assist the patient to maintain optimal functioning • Counsel and teach the patient and patient's family • Use nursing care to achieve therapeutic goals for the patient • Apply correct technique in administering patient care • Initiate necessary lifesaving measures in emergencies • Provide the care needed by the patient to achieve health goals • Enable the patient to achieve self-care and independence • Supervise and check the work of other health care providers • Record and exchange information in verbal and written reports
Evaluating— determining the extent to which nursing care has achieved its goals	• Compare actual outcomes with the expected outcomes of therapy • Investigate compliance with prescribed therapy • Record the patient's response to care • Change the care plan and reorder priorities as indicated

c. Organize and schedule study and review sessions to prevent last-minute cramming

d. Take all National League for Nursing (NLN) examinations offered; these provide realistic practice for NCLEX-RN

e. Consider taking an NCLEX-RN review course to prepare for the examination and become familiar with the test procedure

f. Select a review course based on format of the presentation, quality of the written material, opportunity for practice examinations, and policy for retaking the course if necessary

g. Ask instructors or at the bookstore about computer programs or videotapes for examination review

h. Participate actively in the review course; listen carefully and ask questions

i. Identify and concentrate on unclear or confusing content areas

j. Take practice examinations in nursing review books to increase skill and confidence

PATIENT NEEDS

The chart below lists and explains the four classes of patient needs that make up the second category of the National Council Licensure Examination for Registered Nurses.

PATIENT NEEDS	NURSING INTERVENTIONS
Safe, effective care environment	• Promote environmental safety, quality assurance, coordinated and goal-oriented care, and safe and effective treatments and procedures • Provide basic care; reduce risk potential; and promote physiologic adaptation, mobility, and comfort
Physiologic integrity	• Deal with patients having potentially life-threatening or chronically recurring physiologic conditions and patients at risk for developing complications or untoward effects from treatments
Psychosocial integrity	• Deal with stress-related and crisis-related situations • Promote coping skills and psychosocial adaptation
Health maintenance and promotion	• Deal with patients throughout the life cycle • Promote continued growth and development, self-care, integrity of support systems, and prevention and early disease treatment

k. Practice answering multiple-choice questions

l. Review test-taking strategies, such as reading questions and options carefully and focusing on key words

m. Make sure that all arrangements, such as filing the application and paying the test fee, have been made to avoid last-minute worrying

n. Keep all necessary material, such as admission ticket, in a safe place to avoid last-minute searching

o. Plan travel to and accommodations at the test site

p. Prepare equipment and supplies the night before the examination

q. Get adequate rest the night before the examination

r. Arrive at the examination site early

s. Read test directions carefully and follow them exactly

t. Use stress management techniques to minimize anxiety

u. Avoid reading into questions any information that is not there

v. Allow approximately one minute for each question; keep a steady pace

w. Skip difficult questions; note the question number and return to it later; make sure to mark the answer sheet to note skipping of question and to avoid inadvertent wrong answers

x. Make erasures completely; markings may be picked up by the electronic scanner and the question will be marked incorrect

y. If time allows, review answers after completing the examination

z. Don't discuss the test afterward; simply wait for the results

Points to Remember

Every nurse must be licensed to practice.

Each state's or province's nurse practice act contains specific requirements for licensure.

NCLEX-RN is the licensing examination used in all fifty states. It contains approximately 375 multiple-choice questions; each question matches one phase of the nursing process and one type of patient need.

NCLEX-RN test questions are based on health care situations in which decision making is shared by or centered on the nurse or the patient.

A thorough review of nursing knowledge and practice is essential to successful completion of the NCLEX-RN examination.

Glossary

Board of nursing — state-designated agency that regulates licensure

Licensure — legal mechanism that regulates the practice of nursing

National Council Licensure Examination for Registered Nurses (NCLEX- RN) — examination required for licensure; tests the minimum level of competency required in nursing practice

Nurse practice acts — statements developed by a state's or province's board of nursing that broadly define the legal scope of nursing practice to protect the public

Future Considerations

Learning Objectives
After studying this section, the reader should be able to:

● Describe the process of seeking employment.

● Identify strategies to ease role transition.

● Define reality shock.

● Discuss the importance of joining professional organizations.

● Discuss certification, continuing education, and graduate education as means of career advancement.

● List the different types of practice settings for nurses.

● Explain the importance of career planning, malpractice insurance, assertiveness, and networking.

XV. Future Considerations

A. Introduction
1. Introduction to nursing practice begins with the first nursing course in the curriculum
2. As the student progresses, attention turns to licensure and employment (see Section XIV for a discussion of licensure)

B. Employment
1. General information
   a. Identifying personal and professional goals is an important part of seeking employment
   b. Seeking employment is a complex process; making the wrong choice can lead to disillusionment and discontent
   c. Making the right employment choice provides satisfaction and fulfillment, and paves the way to achieving personal and professional goals
   d. Choosing a job is influenced by many factors, including personal circumstances (such as the need to support children, or the need for a flexible work schedule); professional interests (such as pediatrics or community health); willingness to relocate; plans for continuing education; speciality requirements (such as one-year medical-surgical experience for intensive care unit practice); salary; benefits; working conditions; opportunity for advancement; and long-term career goals
   e. Seeking employment should be carefully planned
   f. Seeking employment involves looking for available positions in newspapers and professional journals, at nursing school career days, and through nursing faculty, other professionals, employment agencies, and placement services
   g. Using a résumé to promote a written summary of education, qualifications, and experience helps an applicant give a first impression to a potential employer
2. Qualities to look for in prospective employers
   a. Compatible nursing philosophy and high professional standards
   b. Acceptable method of delivering nursing care
   c. Formal orientation program for recent graduates to ease the transition to the professional role.
   d. Strong commitment to continuing education to ensure continued learning and professional growth
   e. Opportunities for career advancement
   f. Clearly stated salary, benefits, and shift rotation policy
3. Survival strategies
   a. List career goals, preferences for practice, and personal needs to identify requirements for employment

b. Survey job opportunities to identify options
c. Write a letter to each prospective employer; if requesting an appointment, include days and times convenient for telephone or in-person follow-up (see *Sample letter of application*)
d. Proofread letters carefully to remove spelling and grammar errors
e. Type the résumé using one of several standard formats reference (see *Sample résumé,* page 100)
f. When dressing for an interview, remember that a neat, professional appearance makes a favorable first impression
g. Take extra copies of the résumé to each interview
h. Prepare questions about the institution, job, benefits, and other matters of concern before the interview (see *ABC's of a job interview,* page 101)

C. Role transition
1. General information
   a. Role transition occurs between graduation from nursing school and entry into practice
   b. The transition period is exciting and challenging, but also can be difficult
   c. The graduate nurse is energetic and idealistic, but real-life situations and responsibilities can create confusion, frustration, and insecurity

SAMPLE LETTER OF APPLICATION

452 West Street
Freeport, Maine 09877
May 10, 1990

Ellen J. Smith, RN, MS
Director of Nursing Services
Hillside Medical Center
Central City, Maine 09766

Dear Ms. Smith:

I am a senior nursing student at Freeport College, and I expect to receive a BSN degree in June. I am interested in working as a staff nurse on a medical-surgical unit and am particularly eager to begin work as soon after graduation as possible.

In addition to my clinical experience at Freeport College, I have four years' work experience in geriatrics and home care, and I hope to continue working in geriatric care. Details of my work experience are included in my attached résumé.

I would like to schedule an appointment to discuss employment opportunities at Hillside Medical Center. I can be reached by telephone (666-4325) weekdays before 9:00 a.m., or by mail at the above address. I look forward to hearing from you.

Sincerely,

Jane Brown
Jane Brown

SAMPLE RÉSUMÉ

JANE DOE
5749 Park Avenue
San Diego, CA 76554
(757) 652-0087

EDUCATION

Bay Community College, ADN, 1988-1990
San Diego State College, 1984-86, General studies
Conference on Nursing Diagnosis,
Ellwood Hospital, May, 1988

WORK EXPERIENCE

June, 1988 to the present
Baker Nursing Home
85 Main Street
Westville, CA 76548
Title: Nursing assistant
Duties: Provided care to geriatric patients, including
bathing, transfer, and assistance with meals.

September, 1984 to June, 1988
River Insurance Company
87 Pikeway Road Deaver, CA 76548
Title: Part-time clerk-typist
Duties: Typed reports, policies, and bills.

VOLUNTEER EXPERIENCE

Deaver Children's Rehabilitation Center
Deaver, CA 76548
Volunteer in the children's play therapy group once a
week for three hours. Assisted children with games,
arts and crafts, and music.

COMMUNITY ACTIVITIES

Member, St. Edward's Church Chorale
Member, Beechwood Tennis Team

REFERENCES

Mrs. Judy Wood
(707) 888-6543
Assistant Dean for Nursing
Bay Community College
Easton, CA 87665

Miss Marguerite Daley
(707) 654-3299
Director of Nursing
Baker Nursing Home
85 Main Street
Westville, CA 76548

Mrs. Barbara Elly
(707) 654-8765
Director of Volunteers
Deaver Children's Rehabilitation Center
6098 Ocean Avenue
Deaver, CA 76548

ABC'S OF A JOB INTERVIEW

 PRELIMINARIES

Before any interview, take these steps:
- Respond to an employer's ad — send a cover letter and résumé to the prospective employer.
- Ask for a personal appointment with the director of nursing or whoever is in charge of hiring.
- Practice the interview. Rehearse the answers to foreseeable questions about your education, nursing experience, reason for changing jobs or leaving a previous job, your duties in the last job, and nursing philosophy.
- Be prompt on the day of the interview; arrive 10 minutes ahead of the scheduled time, if possible.
- Dress conservatively; be neatly groomed.

B **WHAT TO DO**

Upon entering the interviewer's office, follow these tips:
- Stand until the interviewer suggests sitting.
- Place any personal belongings on a chair or on the floor.
- Address the interviewer as Ms. or Mr. unless the person suggests otherwise.
- Don't slouch or fidget; sit upright and be attentive.
- Don't chew gum or smoke cigarettes.
- Answer the interviewer's questions with confidence.

 WHAT TO ASK

To evaluate the job and the hospital, ask about the following:
- patient-care assignments
- staffing policies
- advancement opportunities
- continuing education
- salary
- working conditions and work shifts
- employee benefits.

    d. The conflict between idealism and realism results in "reality shock" (see Section D)

    e. The graduate nurse cares for more than 2 or 3 patients, cannot seek assistance from an instructor, and discovers that practice is different from theory

    f. Conflict may occur between employer expectations and a recent graduate's abilities

       g. Conflicts with family and friends may exacerbate feelings of inadequacy and powerlessness

       h. The transition can be a period of growth and renewed self-confidence

2. Survival strategies

       a. Begin self-assessment toward the end of the education program; assess theoretical knowledge, skill proficiency and efficiency, and self-awareness

       b. Talk with nurse recruiters and other nursing personnel to learn about employer expectations

       c. Learn as much about the new employer as possible; for example, participate in orientation programs and talk to other employees

       d. Develop a support network that includes experienced staff members and other recent graduates to discuss feelings and frustrations

       e. Periodically assess capabilities, strengths, and weaknesses; work to improve weak areas

       f. Set goals and work to achieve them

       g. Ask for help; question unclear procedures or policies

       h. Use time-management skills effectively

       i. Seek support and guidance from the unit supervisor, unit manager, or team leader; communicate needs and ideas

       j. Use stress-management techniques

       k. Be assertive

D. Reality shock

1. General information

       a. *Reality shock* describes the experience of adjusting to the professional role after graduation

       b. Problems arise when a new graduate's values and self-concept clash with an employer's expectations of a staff nurse

       c. Adaptation to a new role requires time to reorder values and beliefs

       d. Transition to a new role occurs in four phases: the honeymoon phase, shock or rejection, recovery, and resolution

       e. In the *honeymoon phase* the new graduate is happy, excited, and enthusiastic about work

       f. The honeymoon phase gives way to *shock or rejection* when the new graduate feels disillusioned with nursing

       g. With time, the new graduate moves to *recovery* and is able to regain perspective and meet work demands

       h. A new graduate eventually reaches *resolution*, and either adapts and reconciles school and work values, or changes jobs in an attempt to overcome frustration

       i. Not every new graduate experiences every stage of reality shock, but all experience some aspect when adjusting to the new role

2. Survival strategies

       a. Expect a period of discomfort; allow time to grow to avoid feelings of frustration and inadequacy

     b. Take the initiative; make career and professional choices rather than becoming a victim of circumstance

     c. Seek support, guidance, and reassurance from trusted and admired colleagues

     d. Be flexible; let go of unimportant school values and retain those that are critical to growth and self-esteem

     e. Join the state nurses' association and other professional groups that provide support systems, nurture a professional self-image, and help with personal growth

     f. Discuss feelings of frustration with a supervisor or continuing education instructor

     g. Seek feedback on performance from the unit manager or peers to identify strengths and weaknesses and improve skills

     h. Attend continuing education programs to increase knowledge and proficiency

     i. Adapt work demands and habits to energy level; practice stress-management techniques to prevent burnout

E. Professional organizations
   1. General information
     a. Many organizations for nurses address professional, economic, political, and educational issues (See Appendix B, Professional Nursing Organizations Directory)

     b. The professional organization for RNs in the United States is the American Nurses' Association (ANA)

     c. The American Academy of Nursing is an honorary association within ANA; its purpose is to recognize nurses who have made significant contributions to the profession

     d. The National League for Nursing, an organization for RNs and interested nonnurses, is concerned with nursing education, nursing service, nursing administration, and other health care issues

     e. The American Nurses' Foundation (ANF), a nonprofit corporation, supports research related to nursing

     f. The International Council of Nurses is made up of national nursing organizations; it works with similar organizations around the world to address health care and nursing care issues

     g. Specialty organizations, such as the American Association of Critical-Care Nurses (AACN) and the Association of Operating Room Nurses, address issues specific to areas of practice

     h. Professional organizations establish standards for care in nursing practice and speak for nurses in policy-making forums

     i. Government and regulatory agencies look to these organizations for the profession's stand on public issues related to health, education, and social programs

      j. Membership in a professional organization allows the nurse to participate in shaping public policy

      k. Membership in a professional organization helps the nurse keep up with advances in nursing practice and share information and ideas

  2. Survival strategies

      a. Join the state nurses' association to participate in setting state policy for nursing practice

      b. Join the ANA to participate in ANA activities and receive ANA publications

      c. Join a nursing organization that addresses the concerns of nurses in a particular practice setting

      d. Attend professional conferences and conventions to gain knowledge and maintain enthusiasm for nursing

F. Certification

  1. General information

      a. Certification is the process by which a professional organization formally recognizes the right of a nurse to practice in a particular speciality (see *ANA certified specialties)*

      b. Certification usually is based on a written examination and demonstration of current practice

      c. Certification has professional, but not legal, significance

      d. Some states use certification to identify competency for nurses to practice in an expanded role

A.N.A.-CERTIFIED SPECIALTIES

Clinical Specialist Certification (master's degree required)	• Adult Psychiatric-Mental Health Nursing • Child and Adolescent Psychiatric-Mental Health Nursing • Medical-Surgical Nursing
Nurse Practitioner Certification (requires specific educational program)	• Adult Nurse Practitioner (BSN plus specific program) • Family Nurse Practitioner (BSN plus specific program) • Gerontological Nurse Practitioner • Pediatric Nurse Practitioner • School Nurse Practitioner
Certification in other areas (no educational program requirement)	• Child and Adolescent Nurse • Community Health Nurse • High-risk Perinatal Nurse • Maternal-Child Nurse • Medical-Surgical Nurse • Nursing Administration (BSN required) • Nursing Administration, Advanced (master's degree required) • Psychiatric and Mental Health Nurse

e. ANA certification requires a written examination and demonstration of current practice in a specific area

f. Organizations that offer certification programs include the American College of Nurse Midwives, the American Association of Nurse Anesthetists, and the American Association of Critical-Care Nurses

g. Programs that prepare nurses for specialty practice vary widely: Some can be completed in 6 months; others require a master's degree

h. Requirements for speciality certification vary from state to state

i. Titles used by nurses certified in specialty practice are not standardized and can be confusing

j. Certification is not lifelong; it requires reexamination after a number of years as specified by the professional organization

3. Survival strategies

a. Contact the appropriate professional organization for information about certification requirements and application procedures

b. Learn other nurses' opinions about certification

c. Investigate job-related benefits of certification, such as increased salary or greater opportunity for advancement

d. Prepare for certification examination (see Section X and Section XI for test-taking strategies)

G. Continuing education

1. General information

a. Continuing education (CE) programs are organized learning programs that update nursing knowledge and enhance nursing practice

b. Information obtained through CE programs can be applied to any nursing position

c. CE programs may be lectures, workshops, seminars, symposia, classroom series, computer-assisted instruction, multimedia presentations, planned clinical experiences, or home-study programs

d. CE program providers include hospitals or other health care institutions; colleges; professional organizations, such as ANA and state nurses' associations; national specialty associations, such as AACN and Emergency Nurses Association; national health care organizations, such as the American Diabetes Association (ADA); federal nursing services; and business organizations such as nursing and medical book and magazine publishers

e. CE units are earned when a program is completed

f. The number of units earned is based on the amount of time spent in the program

g. Fifty minutes of participation in the program equals one contact hour; 10 contact hours equals one CE unit (CEU)

h. Continuing education can be voluntary or mandatory

   i. *Voluntary* continuing education allows the nurse to choose programs of interest solely for professional development

   j. *Mandatory* continuing education requires a nurse to earn a minimum number of CEUs for relicensure

   k. The number of CEUs required is specified in the state's nurse practice act

   l. Approximately one-third of the states in the United States require mandatory CE for relicensure

  2. Survival strategies

   a. Identify professional and educational needs and goals to define interest areas

   b. Check the state nurse practice act to determine whether continuing education is mandatory or voluntary

   c. If CE is mandatory, note the number of CEUs required and the time allowed to accumulate them

   d. Get on the mailing list of CE providers to learn about available courses

   e. Check local institutions, nursing service administrations, staff development departments, and professional and speciality organizations for information on programs

   f. Read CE program descriptions; evaluate purpose, objectives, content, teaching methods, and faculty credentials

   g. Make sure the program is approved by an appropriate organization

   h. Determine if program costs are reasonable, affordable, and appropriate for identified needs

   i. Approach employer about possible payment or reimbursement of CE fees

H. Graduate education in nursing

  1. General information

   a. Graduate education consists of education programs that offer specialized advanced degrees

   b. Graduate programs can lead to increased professional responsibilities and career advancement

   c. Graduate education is designed to underscore and advance the professional status of nursing

   d. Graduate education includes master's and doctoral programs

   e. Admission to a master's program requires a bachelor's degree

   f. Additional master's degree prerequisites vary; however, most programs require graduation from an NLN-accredited bachelor's program in nursing, current licensure as a registered nurse, satisfactory undergraduate grade point average, and satisfactory scores on either the Graduate Record Examination or Miller Analogies Test

   g. Master's programs focus on nursing theory, research, issues and clinical specialization; some require additional focus on the nurse's functional role such as clinician, teacher, supervisor, or administrator

    h. Nursing degrees granted at the master's level include master of science in nursing (MSN); master of science with a major in nursing (MS); master's in nursing science (MNSc); master's in nursing (MN); master of arts with a major in nursing (MA); master of public health with a major in nursing (MPH)

    i. The different types of master's degrees reflect institutions' varying curricula and degree-granting powers

    j. Doctoral program prerequisites vary; however, all require a master's degree

    k. Doctoral programs focus on theory and research; they prepare scholarly nurses who can generate and expand nursing knowledge and apply it to the profession

    l. Nursing degrees granted at the doctoral level include doctor of philosophy (PhD); doctor of nursing science (DNSc); doctor of education (EdD); doctor of science in nursing (DSN); doctor of nursing (DN)

    m. The type of doctoral degree granted reflects the program's focus; for example, a PhD in nursing denotes a research-oriented degree for generating new theoretical knowledge through original research; a DNSc degree denotes a practice-oriented degree for generating new clinical knowledge or applying current knowledge to clinical practice

  2. Survival strategies

    a. Identify career goals and determine need for graduate education

    b. Contact professional organizations such as NLN for lists of schools that offer graduate degrees

    c. Investigate programs of interest; review curricula, faculty, facilities, and degrees offered

    d. Ascertain whether program meets needs and goals

    e. Enlist the support of faculty, friends, and family in decision making

    f. Identify conflicts and problems that may arise from pursuing advanced education; make plans to minimize or resolve them

    g. Use time-management and stress-management techniques to facilitate role transition

I. Practice settings

  1. General information

    a. The practice setting is the place where health care is delivered to a patient

    b. Traditionally, the practice setting most closely associated with nursing has been the hospital

    c. Historically, however, most nurses worked outside the hospital; for example, in the 19th century, most nurses practiced in doctors' offices, in patients' homes, or on battlefields

    d. Societal changes, technologic advances, increased consumer involvement in health care, and an emphasis on preventing illness and promoting wellness have changed health care and the settings in which it is delivered (see *Alternative practice settings*)

    e. Factors influencing the nurse's selection of an alternative practice setting include desire for increased independence or change in responsibility; convenient and flexible hours; reduced stress; and attractive salaries, incentives, and benefits

    f. Regardless of the practice setting, the primary focus of nursing care is the patient

    g. Nursing students should consider alternative practice settings when planning for employment after graduation

    h. Certain practice settings require advanced education and experience

    i. Nursing roles, functions, legal liabilities, and responsibilities may vary depending on the practice setting

    j. All nurses, whatever their practice setting, are held accountable to the same nursing practice standards

2. Types of practice settings

    a. Hospitals, including special care units such as critical care, emergency department, and neonatal intensive care

    b. Doctor's office

    c. Outpatient facilities such as ambulatory care centers and women's centers

    d. Community health services such as Visiting Nurse Associations (VNA), public health departments, home health care, occupational health care, school nursing, surgicenters, freestanding emergency clinics, psychiatric outreach programs, and camps

    e. Long-term care facilities such as nursing homes, convalescent centers, residential care facilities, senior citizen continuing care complexes, and rehabilitation centers

    f. Hospice care

    g. Government services, including public health service, armed forces, Veterans' Administration, and Peace Corps

    h. Nursing education, including teaching, educational administration, and research

    i. Independent practice, including private-duty nursing, agency nursing, nurse practitioner practice, publishing, and recruiting

    j. Businesses, including insurance companies and health maintenance organizations (HMOs)

3. Survival strategies

    a. Examine likes and dislikes throughout nursing education to determine interests

    b. Assess personal and professional needs and career goals

ALTERNATIVE PRACTICE SETTINGS

The chart below details how nurses work in four alternative practice settings — schools, industry, community, and business.

PRACTICE SETTING	NURSE'S RESPONSIBILITIES
School	• Provides nursing care for sick or injured students • Gives first aid in emergencies • Gives students medications (when authorized by the school doctor) • Helps school doctor give routine examinations • Gives annual screening tests — for example, vision, audiometry, and scoliosis tests — and refers students for further testing or treatment when appropriate • Counsels parents and students • Meets with teachers and other staff members about health problems and health education programs • Enforces state immunization policies for school-age children • Visits sick or injured students at home when necessary • Helps identify and meet special needs of handicapped students
Industry (Occupational Health)	• Provides nursing care for sick or injured employees • Gives first aid in emergencies • Performs medical screening tests or helps doctor perform them • Refers sick or injured employees for appropriate treatment • Counsels employees on health matters • Meets with employer regarding health-related issues • Develops and maintains employee medical records • Maintains records for government agencies such as workmen's compensation agencies, the Occupational Safety and Health Administration, and state or federal labor and health departments • Alerts employer to potential health and safety hazards
Community (Home Health)	• Provides nursing care for community patients; visits sick or injured persons in their homes • Refers patients for treatment, when appropriate • Coordinates patient care services with patient, family, and health care staff • Communicates regularly with patients, families, and other health care staff • Supervises home health aides and other community health workers • Helps in agency planning by helping to define and set priorities • Works with other professionals to identify and evaluate threats to community health, such as communicable diseases

continued

ALTERNATIVE PRACTICE SETTINGS continued

PRACTICE SETTING	NURSE'S RESPONSIBILITIES
Community (Home Health) (continued)	• Works with private-sector community health workers, such as visiting nurses • Works as a public school nurse, when needed
Business (Insurance Company)	• Screens incoming patients by reviewing records and assessing insurance claims • Helps assess an insurance claim by talking to the patient, his doctor, his family, and his employer • Helps design patient care plans, including medical, nursing, social service, and payment goals • Monitors the patient's progress and prognosis by talking to the patient and his doctors • Helps coordinate medical, rehabilitation, and other services to improve the insured patient's physical condition so he can return to work • Supervises other nursing case reviewers • Develops and maintains insurance company records

    c. Talk with nurses who work in alternative practice settings to get first-hand information

    d. Contact professional organizations for information about alternative practice settings

    e. Determine the need for additional education and, if necessary, make appropriate plans

    f. Investigate legal liabilities associated with alternative practice settings

    g. Develop specific skills required for alternative practice settings; for example, assertiveness, independent decision making, and flexibility

    h. Attend continuing education programs on alternative practice settings

J. Career planning
  1. General information
    a. Nursing offers many satisfying career options
    b. Career planning involves making short- and long-term plans to achieve career goals
    c. Establishing and achieving short-term goals increases the likelihood of achieving long-term goals
    d. Identifying strengths, weaknesses, and interests is essential to career planning
    e. Career planning demands self-awareness and self-initiated change
    f. Career planning allows control, minimizes dissatisfaction, and enhances self-confidence

2. Survival strategies
    a. Identify strengths and weaknesses
    b. Identify skills and personality traits that contribute to strengths
    c. Identify career areas where these skills and traits would be valuable
    d. Choose a career path that incorporates strengths and, if possible, helps overcome weaknesses
    e. Identify resources to help meet short-term goals
    f. Set realistic time limits in which to meet short-term goals
    g. Establish objective standards to judge successful completion of each short-term goal
    h. Take risks; learn new skills and tasks necessary to meet and exceed short- and long-term goals

K. Malpractice insurance
1. General information
    a. Malpractice is professional negligence, such as wrongful conduct, improper discharge of duties, or failure to meet standards of care, that results in harm to another person
    b. Since the 1970s, the number of malpractice lawsuits filed against nurses has increased dramatically
    c. Patients are increasingly aware of their right to receive quality health care and increasingly willing to fight for it
    d. Nurses can protect themselves from malpractice lawsuits by providing the best possible care according to the highest professional standards, understanding and protecting patients' rights, and understanding their own rights and how to safeguard them
    e. Unfortunately, no nurse is perfect and errors do occur
    f. Malpractice insurance (professional liability insurance) provides protection from the financial consequences of certain professional errors
    g. In the event of a lawsuit, the insurer also provides attorneys for legal representation during litigation
    h. A student nurse may be covered by the institution's liability policy or may be required to purchase a liability insurance policy from the school at a nominal fee
    i. Health care institutions are not required to provide malpractice insurance for employees; most do, however, because an employer is usually liable for an employee's errors under the doctrine of *respondeat superior* (Latin for "Let the master answer")
    j. Nevertheless, each nurse should carry professional liability insurance
    k. A nurse in advanced practice roles, such as nurse midwife, nurse anesthetist and nurse practitioner, may require professional liability insurance specific to those functions
2. Types of professional liability policies
    a. Occurrence policy: protects against any error of omission or commission that occurs during a policy period, even if a claim is not made until after the policy expires

   b. Claims-made policy: protects against claims made during the policy period only
3. Survival strategies
   a. When seeking employment, check with the nurse recruiter about the institution's policy on liability coverage for employees
   b. Contact professional organizations to see if they offer policies or can recommend insurance companies
   c. Check professional nursing journals for advertisements for policies
   d. Determine personal needs based on the area of practice
   e. Decide whether an occurrence or claims-made policy best fits needs
   f. Compare features of several professional liability policies
   g. Evaluate policies for options such as coverage when subordinates are negligent; coverage for misuse of equipment, errors in medication administration, or errors in reporting or recording care; coverage for failing to teach patients properly; coverage in case the institution countersues; and coverage for professional services performed in an emergency outside the employment setting
   h. Make sure policy limits are extensive enough to protect assets
   i. Make sure policy is affordable
   j. Select and purchase policy

L. Assertiveness
1. General information
   a. Historically, nursing—because of its handmaiden image and prevalent social customs—has taken a subservient role
   b. This discouraged nurses from being direct and open when confronting professional issues
   c. Today's nurses are striving to abandon the handmaiden image; one way to do so is through assertiveness
   d. Assertive behavior is based on self-confidence; it allows direct and honest expression of needs, opinions, and feelings
   e. Assertiveness involves a balance between nonassertive (passive) behavior and aggressive behavior
   f. Nonassertive behavior results from feelings of inadequacy and the inability to stand up for one's rights; the nonassertive person avoids confrontations and unpleasant situations
   g. Aggressive behavior is the insistence that one's rights, needs, and feelings take precedence over those of others'; the aggressive person typically is self-righteous and egotistical and blames others for problems
   h. Assertive behavior can be learned
   i. An assertive person stands up for his or her rights but is careful not to infringe on the rights of others
   j. An assertive person expresses feelings and needs clearly, honestly, and respectfully through "I-messages," such as "I feel strongly that...because...."

       k. An assertive person faces problems squarely and suggests solutions

       l. An assertive person's self-confidence promotes recognition of personal leadership abilities

  2. Survival strategies

       a. With the help of friends and classmates, assess personal communication style and others' reactions

       b. Identify passive or aggressive behavior and take steps to change

       c. Observe and learn from others' communication styles

       d. Practice making assertive statements to build self-confidence

       e. Offer constructive solutions to problems instead of criticism

       f. Read books and articles about assertiveness techniques

       g. Attend assertiveness training workshops

       h. Develop a positive self-image

       i. Recognize and have confidence in personal and professional rights

       j. Speak directly and calmly; maintain eye contact with the listener

       k. Use "I-messages," such as "I want," "I need," whenever possible

M. Networking

  1. General information

       a. Networking is a process of developing and using a professional system for support, guidance, and information

       b. Networking helps personal and professional growth

       c. Networking is a way to make contacts and referrals, give and receive feedback and emotional support, and initiate change

       d. Networking can include individuals and groups

       e. Networking can begin while student nurses are in school and continue after graduation

       f. Networking can be done on a small scale, with students in a study group sharing information, or on a larger scale, through membership in professional organizations

       g. Networking relies on active involvement and requires time and commitment

  2. Survival strategies

       a. Assess needs and goals

       b. Be willing to seek help from others and to give help when asked

       c. Develop a positive self-image

       d. Identify persons such as colleagues and friends who already make up a support group

       e. Seek out others with common goals and interests

       f. Participate in group activities to expand contacts and resources

       g. Join professional organizations, such as the National Student Nurses' Association and ANA

Points to Remember

Seeking employment is complex and time-consuming; it requires research and planning, identifying career and personal goals, and presenting one's education and qualifications in the best possible light.

A complete, well-prepared, professional résumé is essential for successful job-hunting.

The transition from student to practicing nurse is exciting, but can be frustrating; the graduate must expect a period of adjustment, and should use communication, time-management, and stress-management skills to ease the process.

Membership in professional organizations can foster professional and personal growth and gives the nurse a voice in setting local, state, or national policy on issues of concern.

A nurse should carry professional liability insurance, even if covered under an employer's policy.

Glossary

Claims-made policy — insurance policy that protects against any error made during the policy period, regardless of when a malpractice claim is filed

Malpractice — professional negligence, resulting from lack of knowledge, experience, or skill, that causes harm or injury to a patient

Malpractice insurance — professional liability insurance; provides protection from the financial consequences of professional errors

Occurrence policy — insurance policy that protects against malpractice claims made during the policy period only

Practice setting — place where health care is delivered to the patient

Résumé — document listing information about education, work experience, awards and honors, and volunteer activities; provides prospective employers with a useful summary of qualifications and accomplishments

Appendices

Appendix A

ACT PEP NURSING EXAMINATION CHART

American College Testing Proficiency Examination Program (ACT PEP) tests are used for advanced placement of students into nursing programs. The Classical Curriculum examinations are organized around traditional nursing content areas such as fundamentals, maternity, and pediatric nursing. The Integrated Curriculum exami-nations are organized around the nursing process, life cycles, and patient spectrum. Content related to nutrition and pharmacology is integrated into both exams; the Integrated Curriculum examinations also integrate content from the arts and sciences. This chart describes the various ACT PEP tests.

TYPE OF CURRICULUM	TEST NAME	DESCRIPTION OF TEST CONTENT AREAS
ADN Traditional	Fundamentals of Nursing	• Terminology, facts, principles, and trends • Nursing process • Nursing practice • Basic human needs • Nursing intervention
	Maternal and Child Nursing	• Terminology, facts, principles, theories, and trends • Familial interrelationships • Nutrition • Pharmacology • Pregnancy periods • Child care and development from birth through adolescence
	Maternity Nursing	• Terminology, facts, principles, theories, and trends • Pharmacology • Nutrition • Familial interrelationships • Pregnancy periods • Newborn child care
ADN Integrated	Commonalities in Nursing Care Area A	• Common nursing and nursing care related to patients' basic health needs in safety, communications and interpersonal relations, comfort, rest and activity, skin maintenance and asepsis, the health continuum, and factors that affect health and illness • Knowledge and understanding of technical vocabulary, anatomy, physiology, emotional and physical development, nutrition, and pharmacology

continued

ACT PEP NURSING EXAMINATION CHART   continued

TYPE OF CURRICULUM	TEST NAME	DESCRIPTION OF TEST CONTENT AREAS
ADN Integrated *(continued)*	Commonalities in Nursing Care Area B	• Common nursing problems and nursing care related to patients' basic health needs in nutrition, elimination, oxygenation, and fluid and electrolyte balance. • Knowledge and understanding of technical vocabulary, anatomy, physiology, emotional and physical development, and pharmacology.
	Differences in Nursing Care	• Health care problems commonly encountered by the associate degree nurse. • Routine and specific manifestations of these problems and the nursing care actions properly associated with them. • Acute and long-term problems of medical, surgical, psychiatric, obstetric, and pediatric patients. • Knowledge of technical vocabulary, anatomy and physiology, emotional and physical development, pharmacology, and nutrition.
	Differences in Nursing Care Area A	• Nursing care related to oxygenation and normal and abnormal cell growth.
	Differences in Nursing Care Area B	• Nursing care related to behavioral responses and endocrine and regulatory mechanisms.
	Differences in Nursing Care Area C	• Nursing care related to infection, tissue trauma, and neuromuscular dysfunctions.
	Occupational Strategies in Nursing	• Roles and functions of the associate degree nurse as a contributor to nursing practice within the legal limits of the profession. • The historical perspectives of nursing, the health team, and the nursing team, and the legal guidelines to nursing practice within the context of the history and the current framework of the health care delivery system. • Knowledge and understanding of how licensure, nursing organizations, and education influence the technical nurse's function, as well as ethical guidelines for nursing practice.
BSN Traditional	Psychiatric and Mental Health Nursing	• Terminology, principles, and dynamics • Family development • Personality development • Psychopathology • Nursing intervention • Nursing evaluation

ACT PEP NURSING EXAMINATION CHART continued

TYPE OF CURRICULUM	TEST NAME	DESCRIPTION OF TEST CONTENT AREAS
BSN Traditional (continued)	Adult Nursing	• Physiological, psychological, and sociological aspects of regulatory response mechanisms • Response to stress • Irreversible physiological dysfunction
	Maternal and Child Nursing (baccalaureate degree)	• Physiology and pathophysiology of maternal and child nursing • Theoretical framework of family functioning • Application of the nursing process to practical situations
BSN Integrated	Professional Strategies, Nursing	• Understanding of the professional role. • Professional practice and the health care delivery system. • Development of the nursing program. • Professional organizations, evolution of nursing practice and education, and standards for nursing practice.
	Health Support: Area I	• Patterns that influence wellness and potential barriers to wellness • Use of the nursing process to support the health of the individual, family, and community throughout the life cycle • Patterns of activity, developmental patterns, environment, and the interrelationship of patterns.
	Health Support: Area II	• Patterns that place the individual, family, and community at risk for major health problems, including nutrition, problems of pregnancy, mental illness, cardiovascular and pulmonary diseases, accidents, neoplasms, infections and communicable diseases, and birth defects and genetic problems. • Use of the nursing process to support the health of the patient throughout the life cycle. • Disruptions in activities, nutritional and dietary patterns, developmental patterns, environment, and interrelationships of patterns.
	Health Restoration: Area I	• Interrelationship between the nursing process and changes in the individual, family, and community system. • Nursing process as a framework for assisting patient adaptation to change in a way that promotes restoration, palliation, and rehabilitation.

continued

ACT PEP NURSING EXAMINATION CHART continued

TYPE OF CURRICULUM	TEST NAME	DESCRIPTION OF TEST CONTENT AREAS
BSN Integrated *(continued)*		• Biopsychosocial alterations in response to stressors associated with cardiovascular, respiratory, and autoimmune problems; neoplasms; accidents; and endocrine and metabolic disorders.
	Health Restoration: Area II	• Interrelationship between the nursing process and changes in the individual, family, and community system. • Nursing process as a framework for assisting patient adaptation to change in a way that promotes restoration, palliation, and rehabilitation. • Biopsychosocial alterations in response to stressors associated with mental illness, neurological and sensory disorders, inflammations, infections, and communicable diseases, complications of pregnancy and the high-risk neonate, birth defects and genetic problems, malnutrition, and ecological crises.

Appendix B

PROFESSIONAL NURSING ORGANIZATIONS DIRECTORY

INTERNATIONAL

International Council of Nurses and the Florence Nightingale International Foundation
P.O. Box 42
1211 Geneva 20, Switzerland

Pan American Health Organization WHO Regional Office for the Americas
525 23rd St., NW
Washington, DC 20037

World Health Organization
Avenue Appia
1211 Geneva 27, Switzerland

CANADA
National Organization

Canadian Nurses Association
50 The Driveway
Ottawa, Ont. K2P 1E2

Provincial Professional Associations/Boards of Nursing

ALBERTA
Alberta Association of Registered Nurses
10256 112th St.
Edmonton, Alta. T5K 1M6

Alberta Nursing Assistants Registration Board
10030 107th St., 8th Floor
Edmonton, Alta. T5J 3E4

BRITISH COLUMBIA
Registered Nurses' Association of British Columbia
2855 Arbutus St.
Vancouver, B.C. V6J 3Y8

British Columbia Council of Practical Nurses
3405 Willingdon Ave.
Burnaby, B.C. V5G 3H4

MANITOBA
Manitoba Association of Registered Nurses
647 Broadway
Winnipeg, Man. R3C 0X2

Manitoba Association of Licensed Practical Nurses
1-130 Marion
Winnipeg, Man. R2H 0T4

NEW BRUNSWICK
New Brunswick Association of Registered Nurses
231 Saunders St.
Fredericton, N.B. E3B 1N6

Association of New Brunswick Registered Nursing Assistants
39 Coventry Crescent
Fredericton, N.B. E3B 4P4

NEWFOUNDLAND
Association of Registered Nurses of Newfoundland
55 Military Rd., P.O. Box 4185
St. John's, N.F. A1C 6A1

NORTHWEST TERRITORY
Northwest Territory Registered Nurses' Association
Box 2757
Yellowknife, N.W.T. X0E 1H0

NOVA SCOTIA
Registered Nurses' Association of Nova Scotia
6035 Coburg Rd.
Halifax, N.S. B3H 1Y8

Nova Scotia Board of Registration for Nursing Assistants
5614 Fenwick St.
Halifax, N.S. B3H 1P9

ONTARIO
College of Nurses of Ontario
600 Eglinton Ave. E.
Toronto, Ont. M4P 1P4

Registered Nurses' Association of Ontario
33 Price St.
Toronto, Ont. M4W 1Z2

PRINCE EDWARD ISLAND
Association of Nurses of Prince Edward Island
41 Palmers Lane
Charlottetown, P.E.I. C1A 5V7

continued

PROFESSIONAL NURSING ORGANIZATIONS DIRECTORY continued

CANADA
Provincial Asssociations continued

Prince Edward Island Licensed Nursing Assistants Association
P.O. Box 1253
Charlottetown, P.E.I. C1A 7M8

QUEBEC
Order of Nurses of Quebec
4200 Dorchester Blvd. W.
Montreal, Que. H3Z 1V4

Professional Corporation of Nursing Assistants of Quebec
1980 Sherbrook West, Rm. 920
Montreal, Que. H3H 1E8

SASKATCHEWAN
Saskatchewan Registered Nurses' Association
2066 Retallack St.
Regina, Sak. S4T 2K2

YUKON TERRITORY
Yukon Nurses Society
Box 5371
Whitehorse, Yuk. Y1A 4Z2

UNITED STATES
National Organizations

Alpha Tau Delta National Fraternity for Professional Nurses
489 Serento Circle
Thousand Oaks, CA 91360

American Association of Colleges of Nursing
11 DuPont Circle, Suite 430
Washington, DC 20036

American Association of Critical-Care Nurses
P.O. Box C-19528
Irvine, CA 92660

American Association of Nephrology Nurses and Technicians
505 N. Tustin, Suite 219
Santa Ana, CA 92705

American Association of Neurosurgical Nurses
625 N. Michigan Ave., Suite 1519
Chicago, IL 60611

American Association of Nurse Anesthetists
111 E. Wacker Dr., Suite 929
Chicago, IL 60601

American Association of Occupational Health Nurses, Inc.
575 Lexington Ave.
New York, NY 10022

American Cancer Society
777 3rd Ave.
New York, NY 10017

American College of Nurse-Midwives
1012 14th St., NW, Suite 801
Washington, DC 20005

American Heart Association
7320 Greenville Ave.
Dallas, TX 75231

American Holistic Nurses' Association
P.O. Box 116
Telluride, CO 81435

American Hospital Association Division of Nursing
840 N. Lake Shore Dr.
Chicago, IL 60611

American Nurses' Association American Nurses' Foundation
2420 Pershing Rd.
Kansas City, MO 64108

American Public Health Association
1015 15th St., NW
Washington, DC 20005

American Red Cross
17th & D St., NW
Washington, DC 20006

American Society for Nursing Service Administrators, American Hospital Association
840 N. Lake Shore Dr.
Chicago, IL 60611

Association of Operating Room Nurses
10170 E. Mississippi Ave.
Denver, CO 80231

Association of Pediatric Oncology Nurses
Pacific Medical Center
P.O. Box 7999
San Francisco, CA 94120

Association for Practitioners in Infection Control
1557 N. Pinecrest Rd.
Wichita, KS 67208

PROFESSIONAL NURSING ORGANIZATIONS DIRECTORY   continued

UNITED STATES
National Organizations continued

Association of Rehabilitation Nurses
2506 Gross Point Rd.
Evanston, IL 60201

Catholic Health Association of the U.S.
1438 S. Grand Blvd.
St. Louis, MO 63134

Emergency Nurses Association
666 N. Lakeshore Dr., Suite 1729
Chicago, IL 60611

Gay Nurses Alliance
P.O. Box 1105
Brownsville, TX 78520

Intravenous Nurses Society
87 Blanchard Rd.
Cambridge, MA 02138

National Association of Hispanic Nurses
4359 Stockdale
San Antonio, TX 78233

National Association of Nurse Recruiters
111 E. Wacker Dr., #600
Chicago, IL 60601

National Association of Orthopaedic Nurses, Inc.
N. Woodbury Rd.
Box 56
Pitman, NJ 08071

National Association of Pediatric Nurse Associates and Practitioners
N. Woodbury Rd.
Box 56
Pitman, NJ 08071

National Association of School Nurses
7706 John Hancock Lane
Dayton, OH 45459

National Black Nurses Association, Inc.
425 Ohio Building
175 S. Main St.
Akron, OH 44308

National Council of State Boards of Nursing
303 E. Ohio, Suite 2010
Chicago, IL 60611

National Federation of Licensed Practical Nurses, Inc.
888 7th Ave.
New York, NY 10019

National League for Nursing
10 Columbus Circle
New York, NY 10019

National Male Nurse Association
2308 State St.
Saginaw, MI 48602

National Nurses Society on Alcoholism
P.O. Box 7728
Indian Creek Branch
Shawnee Mission, KS 66207

National Student Nurses' Association, Inc.
10 Columbus Circle
New York, NY 10019

Nurses Association of the American College of Obstetricians and Gynecologists
600 Maryland Ave., SW, Suite 200 E
Washington, DC 20024

Nurses Christian Fellowship
233 Langdon St.
Madison, WI 53703

Nurses Consultants Association
1507 Parkridge
Arlington, TX 76012

Nurses Educational Fund
10 Columbus Circle
New York, NY 10019

Nurses House, Inc.
60 W. 42nd St., Rm. 1616
New York, NY 10165

Oncology Nursing Society
1016 Greentree Rd.
Pittsburgh, PA 15220-3125

Orthopedic Nurses Association
1938 Peachtree Rd., NW
Atlanta, GA 30309

continued

PROFESSIONAL NURSING ORGANIZATIONS DIRECTORY continued

UNITED STATES
National Organizations continued

Sigma Theta Tau
National Honor Society of Nursing
1100 W. Michigan St.
Indianapolis, IN 46223

The Society for Nursing History
Nursing Education Dept.
Box 150
Teachers College
Columbia University
New York, NY 10027

State Professional Associations

Alabama State Nurses Association
360 N. Hull St.
Montgomery, AL 36197

Alaska Nurses Association
237 E. 3rd Ave.
Anchorage, AK 99501

Arizona Nurses Association
1850 E. Southern Ave., Suite 1
Tempe, AZ 85282

Arkansas State Nurses Association
117 S. Cedar St.
Little Rock, AR 72205

California Nurses Association
1855 Folsom St., Rm. 670
San Francisco, CA 94103

Colorado Nurses Association
5453 E. Evans Place
Denver, CO 80222

Connecticut Nurses Association
1 Prestige Dr.
Meriden, CT 06450

Delaware Nurses Association
2644 Capital Trail, Suite R
Newark, DE 19711

District of Columbia Nurses
Association
5100 Wisconsin Ave., NW, Suite 306
Washington, DC 20016

Florida Nurses Association
Box 6985
Orlando, FL 32853

Georgia Nurses Association
1362 Peachtree St., NW
Atlanta, GA 30309

Hawaii Nurses Association
677 Ala Moana, Suite 607
Honolulu, HI 96813

Idaho Nurses Association
1134 N. Orchard #8
Boise, ID 83706

Illinois Nurses Association
20 N. Wacker Dr., Suite 2520
Chicago, IL 60606

Indiana State Nurses Association
2915 N. High School Rd.
Indianapolis, IN 46224

Iowa Nurses Association
215 Shops Bldg., Rm. 215
Des Moines, IA 50309

Kansas State Nurses Association
820 Quincy St., Rm. 520
Topeka, KS 66612

Kentucky Nurses Association
P.O. Box 8342
Station E
1400 S. 1st St.
Louisville, KY 40208

Louisiana State Nurses Association
712 Transcontinental Dr.
Metairie, LA 70004

Maine State Nurses Association
P.O. Box 2240
Augusta, ME 04330

Maryland Nurses Association
5820 Southwestern Blvd.
Baltimore, MD 21227

Massachusetts Nurses Association
376 Boylston St.
Boston, MA 02116

Michigan Nurses Association
120 Spartan Ave.
East Lansing, MI 48823

Minnesota Nurses Association
1821 University Ave., Suite 152
St. Paul, MN 55104

Mississippi Nurses Association
135 Bounds St., Suite 100
Jackson, MS 39206

PROFESSIONAL NURSING ORGANIZATIONS DIRECTORY continued

UNITED STATES
State Professional
Associations continued

Missouri Nurses Association
206 E. Dunklin St.
P.O. Box 325
Jefferson City, MO 65102

Montana Nurses Association
P.O. Box 5718
715 Getchell
Helena, MT 59604

Nebraska Nurses Association
941 O St., Suite 707-711
Lincoln, NE 68508

Nevada Nurses Association
3660 Baker Lane
Reno, NV 89509

New Hampshire Nurses Association
48 West St.
Concord, NH 03301

New Jersey State Nurses Association
320 W. State St.
Trenton, NJ 08618

New Mexico Nurses Association
525 San Pedro, NE, Suite 100
Albuquerque, NM 87108

New York State Nurses Association
2113 Western Ave.
Guilderland, NY 12084

North Carolina Nurses Association
Box 12025
Raleigh, NC 27605

North Dakota State Nurses Association
212 N. 4th Square
Bismarck, ND 58501

Ohio Nurses Association
4000 E. Main St.
P.O. Box 13169
Columbus, OH 43213

Oklahoma Nurses Association
6414 N. Santa Fe, Suite A
Oklahoma City, OK 73116

Oregon Nurses Association
9730 SW Capitol Highway, Suite 200
Portland, OR 97219

Pennsylvania Nurses Association
P.O. Box 8525
Harrisburg, PA 17105

Puerto Rico Board of Nurse Examiners
800 Roberto H. Todd Ave.
Stop 18, Santurce, PR

Rhode Island State Nurses Association
345 Blackstone Blvd.
H.C. Hall Bldg. (South)
Providence, RI 02906

South Carolina Nurses Association
1821 Gadsden St.
Columbia, SC 29201

South Dakota Nurses Association
1505 S. Minnesota, Suite 6
Sioux Falls, SD 57105

Tennessee Nurses Association
1720 West End Bldg., Suite 400
Nashville, TN 37203

Texas Nurses Association
300 Highland Mall Blvd., Suite 504
Austin, TX 78752

Utah Nurses Association
1058A 900 South
Salt Lake City, UT 84105

Vermont State Nurses Association
500 Dorset St.
South Burlington, VT 05401

Virginia Nurses Association
1311 High Point Ave.
Richmond, VA 23230

Washington State Nurses Association
83 S. King St., Suite 500
Seattle, WA 98104

West Virginia Nurses Association
512 "D" St.
South Charleston, WV 25303

Wisconsin Nurses Association
6117 Monona Dr.
Madison, WI 53713

Wyoming Nurses Association
Majestic Bldg., Rm. 305
1603 Capitol Ave.
Cheyenne, WY 82001

Appendix C

SAMPLE NCLEX-RN QUESTIONS

The following sample questions illustrate how National Council Licensure Examination for Registered Nurses (NCLEX-RN) test questions are written and coded according to the Nursing Process (NP) and Patient Needs (PN) categories. The correct answer is indicated by an asterisk (*).

Baby Jones arrives in the newborn nursery weighing 5 lb. 5 oz. His mother's history shows polyhydramnios. He displays excessive salivation, with periodic choking, coughing, and sneezing.

1. To which problem should you give first priority?
   1. Fluid volume deficit potential
   2. Ineffective breathing pattern
   3. Alteration in tissue perfusion
   *4. Ineffective airway clearance
   NP: Planning
   PN: Physiologic integrity

2. Baby Jones continues to have coughing and choking episodes with cyanosis. He also exhibits some gastric distention. Which position is correct for Baby Jones?
   1. Supine with head lowered
   2. Horizontal on the right side
   *3. Supine with head elevated
   4. Prone with head elevated
   NP: Implementing
   PN: Physiologic integrity

Andrew Smith, age 18, is admitted to the hospital for diagnostic studies because of generalized seizures. Gross physical findings are within normal limits. His admission orders include seizure precautions.

3. Since Mr. Smith has had generalized seizures, which question can provide important information about him?
   1. Does he get excited easily?
   *2. Does he have an aura?
   3. Does he eat foods high in tyramine?
   4. Does he have ridges on his fingernails?
   NP: Analyzing
   PN: Physiologic integrity

4. Mr. Smith's care plan should include which of the following notations?
   1. Keep padded tongue blades at bedside.
   2. Maintain a cool environment.
   *3. Pad side rails of bed.
   4. Do neuro check q.i.d.
   NP: Planning
   PN: Safe, effective care environment

SAMPLE NCLEX-RN QUESTIONS continued

Janet Rogers is admitted to the psychiatric unit accompanied by her husband. She remains motionless and silent. Mr. Rogers reports that lately his wife has withdrawn from social situations and that for long periods she has remained secluded and immobile in a darkened room.

5. To plan care for Mrs. Rogers, give priority to which of these assessments?
   *1. Is she a danger to herself and others?
   2. When did her symptoms begin?
   3. What does she do for herself?
   4. Can she be induced to give information about herself?
   NP: Assessing
   PN: Psychosocial integrity

6. Assuming that Mrs. Rogers's greatest anxiety results from interpersonal closeness, which of these behaviors would indicate the highest level of response to treatment?
   1. She begins to assume responsibility for her personal care.
   2. She says she has to go home.
   3. She eats in the dining room with other patients.
   *4. She makes eye contact with the nurse.
   NP: Evaluating
   PN: Psychosocial integrity

Index

i refers to an illustration; t refers to a table.